NEW DIRECTIONS FOR EVALUATION
A PUBLICATION OF THE AMERICAN EVALUATION ASSOCIATION

Gary T. Henry, *Georgia State University*
COEDITOR-IN-CHIEF

Jennifer C. Greene, *Cornell University*
COEDITOR-IN-CHIEF

Evaluating Health and Human Service Programs in Community Settings

Joseph Telfair
University of Alabama at Birmingham

Laura C. Leviton
University of Alabama at Birmingham

Jeanne S. Merchant
University of Alabama at Birmingham

EDITORS

Number 83, Fall 1999

JOSSEY-BASS PUBLISHERS
San Francisco

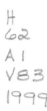

EVALUATING HEALTH AND HUMAN SERVICE PROGRAMS IN COMMUNITY SETTINGS
Joseph Telfair, Laura C. Leviton, Jeanne S. Merchant (eds.)
New Directions for Evaluation, no. 83
Jennifer C. Greene, Gary T. Henry, Coeditors-in-Chief
Copyright ©1999 Jossey-Bass Inc., Publishers, 350 Sansome Street, San Francisco, CA 94104.

Microfilm copies of issues and articles are available in 16mm and 35mm, as well as microfiche in 105mm, through University Microfilms Inc., 300 North Zeeb Road, Ann Arbor, Michigan 48106-1346.

New Directions for Evaluation is indexed in Contents Pages in Education, Higher Education Abstracts, and Sociological Abstracts.

ISSN_0197-6736   ISBN_0-7879-4903-5

NEW DIRECTIONS FOR EVALUATION is part of The Jossey-Bass Education Series and is published quarterly by Jossey-Bass Inc., Publishers, 350 Sansome Street, San Francisco, California 94104-1342.

SUBSCRIPTIONS cost $65.00 for individuals and $118.00 for institutions, agencies, and libraries. Prices subject to change.

EDITORIAL CORRESPONDENCE should be addressed to the Editors-in-Chief, Jennifer C. Greene, Department of Policy Analysis and Management, MVR Hall, Cornell University, Ithaca, NY 14853-4401, or Gary T. Henry, School of Policy Studies, Georgia State University, P.O. Box 4039, Atlanta, GA 30302-4039.

www.josseybass.com

Printed in the United States of America on acid-free recycled paper containing 100 percent recovered waste paper, of which at least 20 percent is postconsumer waste.

Editorial Policy and Procedures

New Directions for Evaluation, a quarterly sourcebook, is an official publication of the American Evaluation Association. The journal publishes empirical, methodological, and theoretical works on all aspects of evaluation. A reflective approach to evaluation is an essential strand to be woven through every volume. The editors encourage volumes that have one of three foci: (1) craft volumes that present approaches, methods, or techniques that can be applied in evaluation practice, such as the use of templates, case studies, or survey research; (2) professional issue volumes that present issues of import for the field of evaluation, such as utilization of evaluation or locus of evaluation capacity; (3) societal issue volumes that draw out the implications of intellectual, social, or cultural developments for the field of evaluation, such as the women's movement, communitarianism, or multiculturalism. A wide range of substantive domains is appropriate for New Directions for Evaluation; however, the domains must be of interest to a large audience within the field of evaluation. We encourage a diversity of perspectives and experiences within each volume, as well as creative bridges between evaluation and other sectors of our collective lives.

The editors do not consider or publish unsolicited single manuscripts. Each issue of the journal is devoted to a single topic, with contributions solicited, organized, reviewed, and edited by a guest editor. Issues may take any of several forms, such as a series of related chapters, a debate, or a long article followed by brief critical commentaries. In all cases, the proposals must follow a specific format, which can be obtained from the editor-in-chief. These proposals are sent to members of the editorial board and to relevant substantive experts for peer review. The process may result in acceptance, a recommendation to revise and resubmit, or rejection. However, the editors are committed to working constructively with potential guest editors to help them develop acceptable proposals.

Jennifer C. Greene, Coeditor-in-Chief
Department of Policy Analysis and Management
MVR Hall
Cornell University
Ithaca, NY 14853-4401
e-mail: jcg8@cornell.edu

Gary T. Henry, Coeditor-in-Chief
School of Policy Studies
Georgia State University
P.O. Box 4039
Atlanta, GA 30302-4039
e-mail: gthenry@gsu.edu

CONTENTS

EDITORS' NOTES

Community-based programming is on the increase in policy sectors such as health and criminal justice. The interest has been spurred by the growing emphasis of public and private funders (mostly foundations) on outcome-based community service programs. As one executive director of a twenty-five-year-old community-based program serving African Americans stated, "They [foundations] know we have and can do it [effectively serve clients], but now they want us to prove it. So, we need help."

This volume of *New Directions for Evaluation* focuses on how to improve approaches to evaluation in community organization settings. These settings can be differentiated from other settings for evaluation by the centrality of the following issues: the assertion of indigenous leadership and control over the program and its evaluation, the intentional access and use of community resources and capacities, and the development of the program explicitly to address perceived needs of community members. Although all community-based programs emphasize these issues, they do so to varying degrees, and thus so do their evaluations. Indeed, the variety of evaluative questions and concerns that arise in community-based initiatives requires not a single community-based evaluation approach, but rather the assessment of varied evaluation approaches for their community context fit. This volume contributes to such an assessment. The practice of community-based program evaluation engages community stakeholders (staff, consortia, partnerships) directly in the process of identifying and assessing problems and solutions through the use of evaluation designs and collaborative, participatory approaches deemed realistic, appropriate, and useful. Both the evaluator and the stakeholders can choose whether the evaluation will serve the community stakeholders or outside stakeholders, or both. The choice has important implications. The evaluator who chooses to serve community stakeholders has a responsibility to facilitate, support, and engage in the problem-solving aspects of these activities rather than accept at face value the definitions of activities, objectives, or criteria that were developed by outside funders and other stakeholders. In this regard the evaluator becomes a collaborator in the enabling process of capacity building (skills, knowledge and resources) and empowerment ideally leading to autonomy and self-determination (Fetterman, 1996; Stringer, 1996; Wallerstein, 1992). We must emphasize however, that we are not proposing a new type of evaluation. On the contrary, evaluation practice in community settings requires an eclectic toolbox of knowledge and skills that will allow evaluators to engage community stakeholders in a flexible yet rigorous evaluation process. It is the process that requires better analysis here, because it is distinctive. This process is time and labor intensive. An evaluator who chooses this work makes a conscious decision to be more personally involved with the community and community-based organizations. This choice will require a closer working relationship with stakeholders at all levels, which will allow for greater input throughout the duration of the evaluation process.

The key difference between community-based evaluation and other types of evaluation lies in understanding and accommodating the unique situations of communities, their leadership, their social and political climates, and their perception of needs, collectively termed the cultural reality of communities.

Traditional human service delivery models are individually or organizationally based, with the emphasis on the technical aspects of the work. In contrast, community-based programs often evolve from the community in response to a mutually recognized need, and the emphasis is on the social, emotional, and political aspects of service delivery. These programs fundamentally focus on the needs or problems of the individual or family from an ecological perspective. Effective programs are those that conceptualize service delivery as a process that begins when the decision is made to provide help and end when all recognize that the help is no longer needed. These programs also recognize that service delivery is influenced by larger economic, social, political, cultural, environmental, historical, and technical factors.

Because service delivery is influenced by the nature, type, and scope of the problem or need, responses, if they are to be effective, must be shaped to address the problems and needs of the individual or family. The problem is not defined by the resources. Community-based organizations that house such programs may often be fragile in terms of funding and leadership. Community leaders themselves often articulate concerns about sustainability.

Finally, community leadership is often less sophisticated technologically; therefore special efforts are required to put useful evaluation tools in their hands.

Community-based program evaluation that respects cultural reality dimensions shares similarities with best practice of general human service delivery evaluation. For example, consultation with stakeholders and the application of stakeholder principles are fast gaining recognition and acceptance in community-based evaluations. Incorporating various views in the design and conduct of program evaluation, a way to ameliorate problems of nonuse and misuse of results, offers clear advantages in community-based evaluation. Community evaluations recognize and facilitate environments of continuous learning and sharing of information, while tailoring their rationale and methods to the reality of community-based programs.

This volume has two aims that are specific to the context and the practice of evaluation in community settings:

To clarify the distinguishing features of the context of community-based programs compared to others. These features influence appropriate evaluation. The distinctive features include the characteristics, special politics, limitations, assets, and needs of such programs.

To describe choices about evaluation practice that are available to the evaluator, the program, and the community in community-based program contexts.

The individual chapters illustrate these two aims. Chapter One, by Joseph Telfair and Laura C. Leviton, offers the voices and perspectives of community-based program leaders regarding the critical characteristics of meaningful community-based program evaluators and evaluations. A salient theme in the chapter is the importance of the evaluator's respect and appreciation for the community context and the program's sociopolitical relationship to it. In Chapter Two, Laura C. Leviton and Russell G. Schuh advance an orientation for the evaluation of community-based programs that incorporates community respect and appreciation. They call this orientation a *discovery capacity*, meaning the continuing capacity of the evaluation to respond to and learn from programmatic and contextual changes and innovations. In Chapter Three, Edith A. Parker, Eugenia Eng, Amy J. Schulz, and Barbara A. Israel, experienced community-based health program evaluators, offer their insights in evaluating changes in community capacity, a goal common to many community-based programs. Reflecting on their experiences, these evaluators describe their lessons learned: the importance of inclusive definitions of community and capacity and of inclusive, participatory evaluation processes. In Chapter Four, Joseph Telfair presents an evaluation prescreening tool, which has been successfully used to match evaluation plans with particular community program evaluation needs, resources, and commitments. Like evaluability assessment, sometimes this match requires reframing or even deferring the evaluation.

Leonard Saxe and Elizabeth Tighe recount in Chapter Five their evaluation of the Robert Wood Johnson Foundation's Fighting Back initiative. This initiative, designed to combat alcohol and drug use, adopts a community-based philosophy. Its evaluation must therefore also respect community contextual uniqueness while simultaneously providing outcome information for national policymakers. Saxe and Tighe present this evaluation as striving for a healthy tension between these national and local views. The final case example, by Rhode Yolanda Crago Alvarez Bicknell and Joseph Telfair, focuses on how to build acceptance of, even commitment to, evaluation in local communities that are engaged in local but externally funded initiatives. Like the Fighting Back example, it highlights tensions between external mandates for evaluation and meaningful local engagement therein. In the final chapter, Abraham Wandersman offers some critical commentary.

References

Fetterman, D. "Empowerment Evaluation: An Introduction to Theory and Practice." In D. Fetterman, S. J. Kaftarian, and A. Wandersman (eds.), *Empowerment Evaluation: Knowledge and Tools for Self-Assessment and Accountability* (pp. 3–46). Thousand Oaks, Calif.: Sage, 1996.

Stringer, E. T. *Action Research: A Handbook for Practitioners.* Thousand Oaks, Calif.: Sage, 1996.

Wallerstein, N. "Powerlessness, Empowerment and Health: Implications for Health Promotion Programs." *American Journal of Health Promotion,* 1992, *6,* 197–204.

Joseph Telfair
Laura C. Leviton
Jeanne S. Merchant
Editors

JOSEPH TELFAIR *is associate professor in the Department of Maternal and Child Health, School of Public Health, and director, Division of Social, Health Services and Community-Based Research within the Comprehensive Sickle Cell Center, School of Medicine, at the University of Alabama at Birmingham.*

LAURA C. LEVITON *was professor in the Department of Health Behavior, School of Public Health, University of Alabama at Birmingham and is now senior program officer for research and evaluation at the Robert Wood Johnson Foundation.*

JEANNE S. MERCHANT *is project coordinator in the Department of Maternal and Child Health, School of Public Health, University of Alabama at Birmingham.*

Interviews with leaders of community-based health initiatives help define meaningful evaluation in contexts in which communities are called on to contribute consent, resources, or participation in program development and research.

The Community as Client: Improving the Prospects for Useful Evaluation Findings

Joseph Telfair, Laura C. Leviton

One of the primary challenges for evaluators of community-based programs is the design and implementation of assessments that are useful and relevant, as well as rigorous (Patton, 1997). Independent of the evaluator's experience level, this can be a difficult process, particularly if the social, political, and technical aspects of the work to be carried out are part of the equation (Herman, Morris, and Fitz-Gibbon, 1987). Working closely with those who are the targets of the evaluation is critical if the challenges are to be adequately addressed. Community-based agency leaders who bring decades of knowledge, experience, and insight are crucial resources who can lay the groundwork for assisting evaluators and other stakeholders in successfully meeting the challenges. This chapter presents the perspectives of these community-based agency leaders through excerpts from interviews that we conducted with four such leaders. The interviews addressed respondents' needs and experiences in commissioning and using evaluations and their vision of ideal evaluation products.

Methodology

The leaders we interviewed were all selected by nomination of professionals and others who have extensive experience with community-based programs and services. Leaders had to meet the following criteria:

Thanks to Jeanne Merchant for her invaluable editorial suggestions.

NEW DIRECTIONS FOR EVALUATION, no. 83, Fall 1999 © Jossey-Bass Publishers

They have worked in community-based settings for at least two decades to ensure that they have experienced the shift from a period of little or no demand for accountability to funders to one of increasing accountability.

They are recognized leaders and innovators in their specific program or service area.

They are recognized leaders in the communities in which they work or contribute.

They have contributed to or participated in the evaluation process for programs or services for which they had responsibility.

They were deemed able to speak freely and honestly about their experiences with evaluation and evaluators.

Another unique characteristic they shared was that they started out working, or continue to work, with agencies that came about in response to a perceived need. Over time, as most other activists do, these leaders have become more expert and sophisticated in their dealings with funders, academics, and evaluators, which has afforded them the skills and insights that are applicable to community-based settings independent of their content, focus of service, or geographic location.

Information was obtained from the leaders in either face-to-face interviews or telephone conference, which we conducted using a structured interview format. The content of the structured interviews was designed to capture each leader's insights and experiences in the following areas:

Needs, which included questions on the types of services, programs, outreach, or advocacy activities that leaders most often needed evaluated; the characteristics that they look for in an evaluator; what is needed to make a sound community-based evaluation; what the leader, his or her colleagues, or clients need to get out of the community-based evaluation experience (what their expectations are); and the ideal evaluation model or approach needed for their unique situation

Experiences, which included questions about how long the leader has been engaged in community-based programs, services, outreach, or advocacy work; their opportunities to participate in the evaluation process (describing how and why they did or did not become involved); and a description of the model or approach to evaluation that has worked best for them or their colleagues and clients

General observations, which included what evaluators who are working or want to work with community clients should know about working with this population

Since many of the content areas overlapped, leaders were given the opportunity to comment in a more in-depth way on areas that may have been mentioned but only briefly discussed. The third content area presented just such a situation.

Finally, content analysis was used in the linking and interpretation of the leaders' comments specific to the content areas.

Profiles of the Community-Based Agency Leaders

Quinton Baker is the director of the Center for the Advancement of Community-Based Public Health in Hillsborough, North Carolina. This center is a grassroots effort that emerged through long-standing community development. He has been involved with community-based programs for close to thirty years.

Here is his explanation of how he gets involved in evaluations of community-based programs:

> I become involved pretty early, as I help to determine the indicators. I have had a problem with evaluations because, frankly, I haven't seen an evaluation being useful. I was not cooperative with the evaluators, say, eight years ago, because I saw them as judging my programs, determining success or failure. Now I know evaluations to be useful for their feedback. They help to inform me if I am on the path to achieve what I want to achieve.

Gladys Robinson and Kathy Norcott work with the Sickle Cell Disease Association of the Piedmont (SCDAP) in Greensboro, North Carolina, where Robinson is executive director and Norcott is program director. The SCDAP is a community-based agency that has provided biopsychosocial services to persons with sickle cell disease for over twenty-five years. Norcott has worked in community-based programs for twenty-two years and likes to get involved in evaluation early in the process to help develop the evaluation tool. Robinson started out writing grants that assisted aging persons twenty-eight years ago and has been working with community-based organizations ever since.

Robinson's experience with community-based evaluation has taught her

> how critical it is to have evaluations of programs like our sickle cell program, because we need to prove ourselves. You see, in my experience, issues like aging, which are broad based, global, and generic, have had the support. But grassroots programs that deal with stigmatized or racial groups, like sickle cell or HIV/AIDS, have always had to fight for their place in society.

Verena G. "Vee" Stalker is a community organizer and advocate who is housed in the Center for Community Health Resource Development at the University of Alabama at Birmingham. She develops and works extensively with social and health initiatives serving poor and rural populations in Alabama and has been involved in community advocacy and development for over forty years. Following are her comments on how evaluation has been useful to her:

> In working with tribes in the West, disenfranchised African Americans, the Red Cross, the U.S. Department of Labor, and the University of North Carolina at Chapel Hill [UNC], among others, I have worked to get into the knowledge base of the area and to defuse the feeling of resentment about evaluating their place.

An example of a project on which I have been working recently is one with Bob and Beverly Cairns of UNC, evaluating the effectiveness of an aggression-reduction program in Wilcox and Perry counties. The project takes place in the school setting and works to keep aggression in check by involving children in activities in which they are interested, such as photography or American jazz. The results have shown that the activities lead to reductions in the rates of aggressive behavior and school dropout. The program is incorporating more traditional learning into the curriculum, such as having a photography student write a paper about a picture he or she took. Thus, evaluation not only demonstrates that this program is successful, but it also suggests positive changes for the future and makes use of local community capacity.

Finally, Ricardo Guzman is the director of the Community Health and Social Service Center (CHASS), a comprehensive community health center that works with the Urban Research Center in southwest Detroit, Michigan. He has been involved in community-based programs for about thirty years. He gets involved with evaluations of community-based programs in this way:

In the vast majority of the projects within the Urban Research Center, I am involved in the planning phase of the evaluation. When the process involves coming to us and allowing us to become a part within the development of the process, we feel positive about it. The evaluation instruments need to be assessed for cultural competency, and for that our input is definitely needed.

When Evaluation Should Be Done

Leaders were unanimous in their opinion that evaluation is needed and appropriate wherever there are broad policy implications of a program. Stalker uses Children's Health Insurance Program (CHIP), an initiative to extend health insurance to all children, as a good example of a program with such implications. The implementation of this program brings to the light many important questions related to evaluation—for example:

- How do you get people enrolled in a timely fashion?
- What does the enrollment process tell you about people who never sign up for Medicaid?
- What happens to the people once they are enrolled? Does it help? Do providers get overloaded?

Stalker described one example of provider overload that is a problem in Alabama. Because Alabama Medicaid pays little in reimbursement to dentists, many dentists cannot afford to provide services to Medicaid-eligible people. So as CHIP brings more children into the dental health care system, the dentists who do see Medicaid patients and are already overloaded will not be able to take on this new influx of consumers. The obvious solution to the problem is to increase Medicaid coverage to dentists in the state. One way to facilitate this political process is to evaluate the current Medicaid dental coverage and what happens as CHIP is implemented. These results could be sent to state dental schools and professional dental associations.

The leaders agree that evaluation is also clearly necessary when programs offer direct services. With direct service programs, evaluation is done to show accountability and specific outcomes. Now, with contact services and education of the general public, evaluation will probably be done in the future to determine if these outreach programs are making an impact.

Those interviewed all stressed that ultimately the only way to be an advocate and to secure social justice for those who need it is to conduct appropriate evaluations. Good advocates need numbers to back up their statements, says Vee Stalker: "For too many years we've just marched on the basis of principle, but without numbers we are not taken seriously." She noted that evaluations need to show why programs work, as well as why they are needed.

Types of Services Where Evaluation Is Most Often Needed

Ricardo Guzman believes that there are two aspects to this issue. One is primary health care, which is basically what CHASS provides. Outcome evaluation for the center's basic services is established and agreed to. The ongoing community-based programs generally have a built-in outcome evaluation component. But for services that the center staff do not normally provide, they end up not having the time, energy, or staffing to handle evaluation. One example is a domestic violence program that recently started in collaboration with several other community-based organizations in southwest Detroit. For this and for any other activity where the center staff write grants that are beyond the scope of normal activity, they need assistance with evaluation. Guzman has noticed that new collaborations, such as the domestic-violence-prevention effort, take time. The center is making linkages with groups in other parts of Detroit where they have not previously worked, "which does not happen overnight," he says.

Quinton Baker gives more insight into the types of programs that most often need evaluation. He needs to have programs that strive for community health improvement evaluated. For instance, for his center's diabetes program, the capacity of the community to address its own issues is of paramount importance and needs to be evaluated. But this kind of evaluation is difficult to do because improved capacity is hard to define, and it is a more long-range goal than are specific services (see Chapter Three on evaluating community capacity). It is important to remember that community-based evaluation needs to be done three to five years after a program is initiated. The reason is that during the course of the program, it is very difficult to take unintended consequences into consideration.

Characteristics of a Good Evaluator

Most of the leaders agreed that good evaluators are not so focused on what they are looking at that they lose their peripheral vision. Evaluators need to be enmeshed in the community and determine what they are trying to accomplish in the context of what else is going on. The leaders believe that there is a tendency for evaluators to become too task oriented, which should be avoided. It is always best to conduct the evaluation in participant-observer, anthropologic terms, because community members seem to respond best to this approach, although incorporating quantitative methods to satisfy most funders is crucial.

The respondents point out that another characteristic of good evaluators is that they will pilot-test any evaluation design with local input first. This has the benefits of demystifying the project and turning community leaders into spokespeople for the program. This builds on the "grapevine" effect, which is important in rural areas because a lot of information is passed from person to person.

The leaders believe that to be successful, an evaluator must have a clear understanding of communities and laypeople. Community leaders must understand what evaluators do, and evaluators need to have that intangible component that makes understanding possible. They must be able to explain the kinds of things that have to be done in evaluations, which are difficult to understand without a context. Even if an evaluator does not have people skills, he or she can get "over the hump" with a good understanding of and value for the community and what it does. Above all, they argue, a good community-based evaluator is willing to interact with community members and leaders on a routine basis, as an integral part of the evaluation process.

Characteristics of a Good Evaluation

Interviewees agree that the community needs to be involved in helping to establish the indicators and priorities of the evaluation. An evaluation must be outside the realm of policing; that is, it should not be seen as auditing a program. Most evaluations need to be participatory. Leaders concur that rigid scientific models without participation do not work well in community evaluations. Ricardo Guzman says, "they tend to turn people off and folks won't buy in." A good evaluation lends itself to community members' being able to interact with the evaluator. Community members from the outset must be part of the process. If the evaluation is participatory, the interviewees say, the process really works.

Ricardo Guzman stresses the need for the evaluation to be culturally competent. He comments on the unique approach that must be taken in AIDS education for predominantly Latina populations:

> Cards were sent to us that we were supposed to distribute to women in the community that depicted very graphic pictures describing how to correctly put a condom on a man. These were designed for the East and West Coasts, and the health professionals were trying to just drop the same techniques into the Midwest. Around here, we use fruit. Using a banana in condom instruction works

very well because people can laugh and relax, and then they are more open to paying attention. If you use an anatomically correct model, a Mexican American woman won't even touch it. These cultural differences are crucial to understand if a program is to work, as well as in program evaluation.

One interviewee pointed out that for an evaluation to be effective, the program being evaluated must have clearly defined goals and services and be working to reach these goals. In other words, says Robinson, "Are you fulfilling some kind of need, and can it be measured"? Second, there need to be people on site who know what it takes to get data packaged. A good evaluation should also let workers know how their role helps the overall effort. It is sometimes difficult for nonprofits to get funding for evaluations, because they get tired of writing grants, and funding is never stable. For this reason, evaluations have been seen as a hindrance in the past. Nevertheless, evaluations have made it possible for Robinson to approach a funding source and be able to show that the program is a good one. "Evaluations allow you to say that with more certainty," she explains, "and have saved us dollars, actually. We have come a long way, and have finally gotten our staff to realize the link between evaluation, its use, and the maintenance of their jobs."

Stalker gives some specific examples of components that always need to be a part of an evaluation of a community-based program:

- Demographics
- Historical organization in the area (often found by searching old theses and dissertations)
- An understanding of the local government and the shadow government (often the real power structure)
- Land usage patterns (in particular, who controls the land and for how long)
- Traffic patterns
- Market patterns
- Where individuals who have to leave the area for something go
- An assessment of the local tax structure (especially regressive tax)
- Knowledge about the local media (making note of any affiliations of the editor and the editorial policy, which also provides information about the shadow government)
- Attitudes of state government on issues like race, the status quo, and economic development

All of these features of a community are an integral part of the success or failure of any program and must be assessed. Stalker believes that in Alabama, regressive attitudes maintain the status quo in many areas. An example is the continued reliance on county governments rather than regional ones. In the past, each county seat was situated so that residents could reasonably get to the county seat and back to their homes before dark on foot or horseback. In the age of the automobile and with the wide availability of telecommunications, such a system is no longer necessary or useful. She believes that the fact that Alabama continues to use county governments allows patronage jobs to sap away resources and subverts regional strength and progress. This is only one example of the way that larger social issues play into the climate that surrounds any program.

What a Community Can Get Out of an Evaluation

All leaders agree that communities can get feedback about their program as a result of community-based evaluation. The evaluation becomes a tool to hold a mirror up to the community so that it can see what it is doing. It also becomes a tool for community members' own empowerment. For example, Stalker's organization conducted a hand-washing program in the schools of Wilcox County, one of the most impoverished areas in Alabama. Her staff did chart audits for infectious diseases, which indicated that sanitation was a big problem. It is really a problem all over the state "because of the fact that this is the South, and many people reside in mobile homes and other types of housing situations that do not have adequate sewerage." The price of adequate sewerage methods is just too great for a lot of people, she says. The lowest-cost solution to the spread of disease was frequent hand-washing.

Rather than simply telling the local residents to wash their hands, Stalker gave the information to school health employees, who then used it to teach hand washing to food service workers and students. Once teachers realized the importance of hand washing, they willingly passed the information on to their students. When the positive results became apparent, the community teachers felt pride in their accomplishments. This pride helped the program persist even after the academics and practitioners were no longer part of the program. The community infrastructure that results from an evaluation is what makes a health initiative truly successful.

Quinton Baker needs to know from an evaluation, "Are we achieving what we want to achieve? And if not, why? Those are the important issues." The evaluation must leave some markers of success or failure in the community. An evaluation needs to codify these issues so that the community learns to evaluate itself. Baker often hears the criticism that communities want to know only the positive results of an evaluation. His response is, "If a community is involved from the beginning, it is open to hearing the negative, especially if it agrees with the indicators."

Is There an Ideal Evaluation Model or Approach for Community-Based Health Programs?

When a program is germinated in a community, the funders should include an evaluator in their initial plans. If the evaluators are brought in after the project has begun, they seem like an alien part of the process. It needs to be clear whom the evaluators work for and to whom they feel accountable. "It should be community first," says Quinton Baker.

Gladys Robinson and Kathy Norcott suggest that a small grassroots organization may have to form a partnership with an evaluator who would be willing to accept a small fee to begin with. They start on a small scale. Internal evaluations need to take place before external evaluations happen.

Many of those interviewed seemed to be less interested in any particular model and more interested in the substantial questions that relate to the evaluator's approach. This underscores the recurrent theme regarding this issue: no one model is perfectly applicable to community-based evaluation. The evaluator's approach to the community is much more important than the type of model to those being evaluated.

What Evaluators Should Know

The interviewees agree that evaluators need to be clear about ownership of the data and must understand the importance of having input and buy-in from both the evaluator and the community. Sometimes, for instance, the community may be very clear about what the program is trying to do, but not very clear about what a program needs to measure. Part of an evaluator's role is to assist the community members in achieving this clarity.

Evaluators also need to recognize that large funding organizations struggle in trying to deal with communities, and that can make the job of the evaluator more difficult. Many large organizations are used to doing things in a hierarchical manner, which does not work very well in community-based programs. Funders often think that working with the local public health department is working with the community; sometimes that is true—but not always. Ricardo Guzman notes that funders now are at least considering community-based programs seriously, and for this reason, an evaluator should keep in mind that a program needs to show scientific, relevant, and measurable outcomes. If the evaluator can facilitate a rigorous evaluation of outcomes, then most funding organizations will be amenable to letting communities set their own agenda.

In communities of poverty or where there are large numbers of people of color, trust is a big issue, says Quinton Baker: "If they do not trust you, they may not tell you the truth, period." An evaluator must allow for a period of trust building. Baker points out that the evaluator will know when trust is there, because the community client will volunteer extra information in an interview. Things do not happen in communities the way that evaluators are taught in academia. If the community members are guarded about information, the evaluator can collect data, but the data will not be accurate. The challenge is for academics and evaluators to be flexible in their methods, depending on the problem in the community.

Conclusion

At the end of each interview, the professionals were asked for closing thoughts they had for potential community-based evaluators:

Quinton Baker

Well, what do you want to have after this? You want to put yourself out of business. That is very hard to deal with. Many programs are chasing dollars to continue to exist, not to do what they *want* to do. If they work out of the framework of needs, which never go away, then they can couple capacity building with services. Community-based evaluation can be done scientifically and rigorously, and without barriers to members of the community themselves.

Gladys Robinson and Kathy Norcott

Evaluators need to understand nonprofits. Evaluators can have other motives, but they need to be open and honest about them. I always ask prospective evaluators what their motives are, besides getting a degree, experience, or something else. If they really do want to help a struggling organization, that's going to get across to whom they want to work for, because human services folks are some of the most intuitive folks around. Evaluators need to be committed and must be honest with the community. Knowing the community is crucial, as well as having an open mind. Preconceived notions have to be done away with. An evaluator needs to listen to the community-based agency and must be aware that the purpose of the evaluation is to help the organization being evaluated. He or she needs to know that primarily we feel responsible to our clients. The future of nonprofits hinges on evaluations.

Vee Stalker

In the end, evaluators have to reframe their methods to take into account up-front issues, like the tax structure, or race relations, or economic development of the area. An evaluator must invest himself or herself in the process and in the community. If he or she can approach the evaluation horizontally, not vertically, the result will be informative, useful, and fair.

Ricardo Guzman

We are all students, and I hope that evaluators, as well as the communities served, would view themselves as learning research principles, techniques, and skills. This way, neither community nor evaluators are starting anew each time an evaluation is initiated.

References

Herman, J. L., Morris, L. L., and Fitz-Gibbon, C. T. *Evaluator's Handbook.* Thousand Oaks, Calif.: Sage, 1987.
Patton, M. Q. *Utilization-Focused Evaluation.* (3rd ed.) Thousand Oaks, Calif.: Sage, 1997.

JOSEPH TELFAIR is associate professor in the Department of Maternal and Child Health, School of Public Health, and director, Division of Social, Health Services and Community-Based Research within the Comprehensive Sickle Cell Center, School of Medicine, at the University of Alabama at Birmingham.

LAURA C. LEVITON was professor in the Department of Health Behavior, School of Public Health, University of Alabama at Birmingham and is now senior program officer for research and evaluation at the Robert Wood Johnson Foundation.

Maintaining a discovery capacity in evaluation promotes better fit between the evaluation and the dynamic, complex contexts of community-based programs. A continuing discovery capacity also fits well with the long-term, systemic changes to which these programs aspire.

The Importance of a Discovery Capacity in Community-Based Health and Human Service Program Evaluation

Laura C. Leviton, Russell G. Schuh

In this chapter we make the case for maintaining a discovery capacity (both qualitative and quantitative) in evaluations of community-based health and human service programs. Discovery capacity was defined by Robert Stake (1975; 1978) as a mechanism to detect new insights and developments in programs. This capacity is essential throughout the formative phases of evaluation, but often it continues to be critical even after summative evaluation is under way. A general case can be made for continued discovery capacity, even in professionally driven or agency-based evaluation (Stake, 1975, 1978). However, it is especially important in evaluating community-based programs for the following reasons:

Community-based programs are often relatively new compared to agency-based or professionally based programs (Leviton, 1994).
Programs continue to evolve, especially community-based programs (Weiss, 1998).
Communities continue to adopt and adapt strategies to suit new circumstances (Rogers, 1983).
Community members' creativity to address program challenges does not cease just because a summative evaluation is conducted (McKnight, 1995).
The theory behind programs in community settings often incorporates a twofold set of assumptions. The two assumptions need to be uncoupled to evaluate such programs adequately and to avoid confusion over evaluation aims and focus.

NEW DIRECTIONS FOR EVALUATION, no. 83, Fall 1999 © Jossey-Bass Publishers

Assumption I is that increasing community capacity will improve efforts to address health and social problems. Community capacities can be defined as the variety of resources, skills, and commitments that community people can bring to the solution of a problem (Clark and McLeroy, 1995; McKnight, 1995). Assumption II is that specific categorical efforts of community-based programs will be effective when they are targeted to specific conditions or problems.

The first assumption may be true or false depending on circumstances. Development of new capacity or expertise is a gradual process for anyone, professional or layperson. At any given time, is expertise sufficient for the purpose? Also, community capacity may be sufficient, but we may not always anticipate exactly which problems will be improved. The second assumption may or may not be true: an ineffective strategy for a problem is likely to be ineffective whether it is implemented by a community or by professionals.

Nevertheless, some interventions clearly are better conducted in community settings with community participation. A discovery capacity can inform us as to which those interventions are. And tying the two assumptions together, what kinds of health and social problems can be ameliorated through community capacity building? To make the special case for a discovery function in community-based programs, we present five evaluations of community-based programs, some of them federally funded and some of them grassroots efforts. The findings from these evaluations will illustrate our points. We then review relevant principles of evaluation and community development and offer examples of the value of continued discovery. Finally, we reflect on the reasons that discovery might be neglected and describe ways in which both discovery and summative evaluation can be accommodated.

Illustrative Programs and Evaluations

The studies that follow are a heterogeneous group. Some of the interventions emerged directly from community needs and initiatives, while others were created directly by nationally known professionals. Both qualitative and quantitative information served the discovery purpose. In all cases, a continuing discovery capacity remains useful.

The AIDS Community Demonstration Projects. One of the earliest multisite evaluations of HIV prevention conducted by the federal Centers for Disease Control and Prevention (CDC), this initiative used a quasi-experimental design in which ten communities were matched on relevant characteristics (CDC AIDS Community Demonstration Projects Research Group, 1999; Guenther-Grey, Noroian, Fonseka, and Higgins, 1996; Higgins and others, 1996; "Community-Level Prevention...," 1996; Simons and others, 1996). The program's aim was to promote consistent condom and bleach use among injection drug users, female sex partners of injection drug users, female commercial sex workers, at-risk youth, and non-gay-identified men who have sex with men. Compared to control communities, intervention in the target communities achieved a 54 percent exposure rate to messages, significantly greater progress toward more consistent condom use, and a significant increase in carrying of condoms by those at risk. (A Web site, http://www.cdc.gov/nchstp/hiv_aids/projects/acdp/acdp.htm, provides a bibliography and complete program description.) This project began with a detailed qualitative discovery process in order to understand the forces at work in maintaining HIV risk behaviors but then shifted to intervention and collection of survey data.

Pilot Project to Provide Mental Health and Community-Based Services to Adolescent and Youth Victims of Violence from Homewood. The Staunton Farms Foundation supports this collaboration between a grassroots neighborhood initiative and units of the University of Pittsburgh Medical Center (Schuh, Marin, Thompson, and Byrdsong, 1997). The formative evaluation, which is ongoing, aims at developing a testable model from pilot activities. The neighborhood organization joined forces with trauma department professionals who often treated teenagers for gunshots, only to send them back to the streets where they were at high risk of being shot again or shooting others. The neighborhood organization identifies teenagers in the emergency and trauma departments and then follows up with them and their parents once they are released, to try to reduce risk of later homicide. This is the first time we have personally witnessed a foundation's funding formative evaluation.

The Heart Attack–REACT Project. In 1994 the National Heart, Lung, and Blood Institute (NHLBI) initiated the REACT study (Rapid Early Action for Coronary Treatment) with a goal of evaluating a community intervention to reduce patient delay time, defined as the period from the onset of heart attack symptoms until a patient's contact with the medical care system. REACT was a four-year, randomized, multicenter collaborative community trial, with five academic study field centers, each affiliated with four communities (Simons-Morton and others, in press). REACT used community organizations, community and media education, provider education, and patient education to convey the message about the importance of seeking help quickly when heart attack symptoms begin.

Like the AIDS Community Demonstration Projects, REACT began with a highly detailed qualitative effort to understand the processes whereby people experience heart attacks, and react to heart attacks in friends and loved ones, and by which medical professionals deal with heterogeneous symptoms, settings, and health care system constraints (Finnegan and others, forthcoming; Leviton and others, forthcoming; Zapka and others, forthcoming). Like the AIDS Community Demonstration Projects, it also moved to summative evaluation mode, for which the report is under review currently (Russell Luepker, personal communication). Follow-up focus groups indicate some important discoveries about the message and the community efforts, which can be found at http://epihub.epi.umn.edu/~react/welcome.html.

The Partners Continuum of Services. This is a collaboration that unites community-based organizations (CBOs) working in Pittsburgh's Hill District, a low-income African American community, with the Mathilda Theiss Child Development Center, located in a satellite clinic of the University of Pittsburgh Health System. It is supported in part by grants from the R. K. Mellon Foundation and the U.S. Department of Housing and Urban Development. This collaborative targets mothers with housing and addiction problems whose children have developmental problems. Through both qualitative and quantitative discovery, formative evaluation is providing insights about collaboration and about public housing environments.

Halloween Arson Prevention in Detroit. This summative evaluation was a serendipitous discovery that grew out of dialogue between community leaders and the federal staff of the CDC's Urban Research Centers (Maciak, Moore, Leviton, and Guinan, 1998). The Detroit Urban Research Center represents a longstanding tradition of partnership between specific Detroit neighborhoods and the University of Michigan School of Public Health. The evaluation was not planned by this partnership, and no professionally driven interventions preceded it. Instead, the multifaceted anti-arson effort was a direct accomplishment of community-based organizations, working with city police and fire departments. It harnessed the efforts of many volunteers, enforced a new youth curfew during Halloween, and pressured for change in the media presentation of Halloween arson. Figure 2.1 illustrates a major finding: the number of Halloween fires declined from the inception of the program in 1985 to 1996. Important data not presented here indicate that the number of fires was stable and high from 1979 to 1984, and that fires at other times of

Figure 2.1. Total Number of Fires Reported During the Three-Day Halloween Period (Oct. 29–31) and Number of Volunteeers Participating in Arson-Prevention Activities, Detroit, 1984–1986

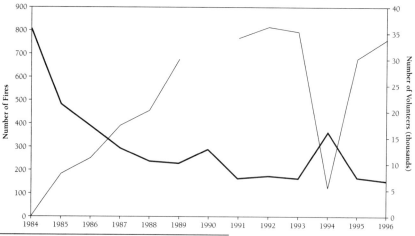

Note: The number of volunteers for 1990 is unavailable.

Source: From Maciak, B., Moore, M., Leviton, L. C., and Guinan, M. "Preventing Halloween Arson in an Urban Setting." *Health Education and Behavior,* 1998, 25, 194–211. Reprinted by permission.

the year remained at a steady state from 1979 to 1996, thus ruling out some potential threats to the validity of the short time series.

Why Maintain a Discovery Capacity in Evaluation?

The linkages among specific activities, mediating processes, and the immediate, intermediate, and ultimate objectives of programs are often poorly understood. Although this is the case for many health and social programs, it is especially true for programs that incorporate different forms of community participation. Here, a discovery capacity is vital to such evaluations.

The Formative Insufficiency Problem. Summative outcome evaluation is conducted prematurely in many programs (Weiss, 1998; Wholey, 1994). We term this typical problem *formative insufficiency,* acknowledging Scriven's (1967) contribution. Programs may suffer from this problem because of untested program theory, implementation problems, or untested evaluation design and measurement. Suchman (1970) originally outlined four stages in program development, which closely mirror the process undertaken in the development and testing of medical procedures:

1. Trial and error, in which developers tinker with a new idea
2. Model development, in which the idea is systematized
3. A formal test of efficacy under ideal conditions
4. A test of effectiveness under flawed, real-world conditions

Unfortunately, research on social programming often curtails or combines some of these stages. Often the model is not fully developed before a field test begins. Wholey (1994) used the term *evaluability assessment* to determine if an intervention or demonstration has reached a sufficient developmental stage to support outcome assessment (See Chapter Four on this issue as well). Lipsey (1985, 1988, 1990) observed that the large majority of evaluation research designs are forced to use a "black box" approach, because the underlying theory or model is so poorly articulated. Reichardt (1994) concluded that outcome evaluations fail to detect results because the programs themselves are not sufficiently well developed to produce them.

Formative Insufficiency in Community Programs. It may be that formative insufficiency is especially problematic for community-based efforts. First, a demonstration program format is frequently used to fund projects involving community organizations. This happens for several reasons:

The organizations may be new, and a demonstration project gives them experience (and gains experience with them).
Community-based programs tend to appear highly specific to a given community and therefore are not appropriate for a general funding announcement.
Community-based projects are frequently innovative concepts and not ready for widespread replication or testing.

Second, there is no such thing as an ideal condition to test an idea in communities, making efficacy tests more difficult. Every community is an open system where situations change and the communities themselves are in flux. Third, the efficacy and effectiveness stages are often combined, because the cost of conducting community-based studies in a rigorous fashion can truly be daunting. Fourth, to the extent that communities are participants in the process, they will continue to engage in trial and error: innovating, inventing, and reinventing the strategies under study.

Formative Insufficiency and Responsive Evaluation. In spite of these problems, we continue to produce evaluations, especially in public health, as though we did understand the underlying theory. Robert Stake (1975, 1978) introduced the concept of responsive evaluation, which can help to address this problem. Responsive evaluation permits an ongoing discovery capacity aimed at identifying emerging themes and new knowledge about programs. (Although Stake advocated the use of qualitative methods and case studies, the discovery capacity is not limited to these techniques, as we will show.) The goal of ongoing discovery is to improve the actual practice of service delivery in programs. In programs that incorporate community participation, we would generally endorse the idea of an increased capacity for discovery, even in circumstances where summative evaluation is under way. The discovery process does not replace summative evaluation when the field is ready for summative evaluation. Instead, it offers many opportunities to enrich understanding of summative evaluation.

Importance of Discovery in Community-Based Programs

The concept of working with community resources and support should not be new to health and human service programs, but it is (Leviton, 1994). Although they were an integral part of the War on Poverty programs, the principles and the know-how of community-based work were somehow lost in the interim. Only in the late 1980s and early 1990s did they reemerge, thanks to the efforts of individuals such as Lawrence Green and Marshall Kreuter (1991). Terms such as *community policing* suggest that other policy sectors have rediscovered the term as well; in general, a new wave of interest has emerged as a result of the communitarian movement in U.S. society (Etzioni, 1993). For reasons we will elaborate in the last section of this chapter, much remains to be discovered about working with communities and about appropriate evaluation of community-based programs (Leviton, Needleman, and Shapiro, 1998).

Community Resources and Community Development. There are many kinds of community-based programs and many functions that community supports can serve, distinctions that are often lost due to rhetoric and lack of experience (Leviton, 1994)—for example:

• Acceptance, as when community leaders are asked to endorse a project or encourage people to participate (Higgins and others, 1996)

- Tailoring of projects to community culture, norms, expectations, needs, and situations (McAlister, 1991)
- Accessing or developing a community's own capacity to address a problem (Clark and McLeroy, 1995; McKnight, 1995; McKnight and Kretzman, 1990)
- Advocacy for services for a client or community (Leviton and Schuh, 1990; Schuh and Leviton, 1991)
- Building political support to address a need (Eng, Parker, and Harlan, 1997)

Communities often continue to develop new strategies to serve these functions, even when a multisite intervention protocol has been agreed to (as in the case of the AIDS Community Demonstration Projects and the Heart Attack–REACT Project). Since the seminal work of Freire (1970) and Alinsky (1972), it has been understood that communities often complete a developmental process and see things differently from those who were not offered that opportunity. Communities at the end of such a process will know more, and know different things, about the nature of the problem, community capacities and resources, the types of activities that are effective locally, and the types of advocacy and political action that are required to solve problems.

These observations are consistent with Herbert Simon's (1970) concept of a continuum in the development of expertise. Agencies are staffed by individuals who have spent years mastering or developing skills in a substantive area. CBOs are composed of individuals whose primary expertise might be understood to be the community and its inhabitants. It has been well established that "experts" see things differently than do novices. In Simon's model, one progresses from novice to advanced beginner, to competent, to proficient, and finally to expert. Research suggests real differences in performance between the stages. Evaluators do not begin with a real proficiency in relating to communities, and community leaders are often at a loss when they first confront program management and evaluation. Communication improves as parties develop greater expertise in their collaborator's substantive area. Sometimes this is termed shared understanding, but it may also be a better vision as people become expert in areas that were originally beyond their realm of experience.

Time Frame to Achieve Community Change. In the rush to conduct summative evaluation, researchers often do not consider that working with communities and developing collaborative efforts takes time—even years—before specific achievements can be identified. For example, participants in the Partners Continuum project attribute much of the group's success to the employment of a Ph.D.-level process counselor whose role is to monitor and protect the health of the collaborative process. Nurturing the process has promoted an unprecedented level of trust and cooperation among the agencies. Once this was in place, the continuum sought its first grant for a specific program. However, in a real sense the collaboration was initiated almost seven years ago. Time was also needed to produce achievements of the Detroit Urban Research Center, which emerged as a result of many hard years of work to establish a relationship between Michigan public health professionals and Detroit community leaders. Such levels of trust and development of community capacity are achieved at a different rate than are specific program goals to address a problem.

Time is also an issue whenever implementation requires that new social networks within communities become engaged in the process. In Figure 2.1, the curve for volunteer participation to combat Halloween arson illustrates the issue. The rate of increase slows only after five or perhaps six years (data are missing for 1990). Similar curves are seen for participation in community-based wellness programs, such as the ongoing program for cardiovascular risk reduction in African American women in Wilcox County, Alabama (Cornell, 1999). Participation in "Cut the Fat" cooking classes kept climbing for months as new community members became involved. Accessing community networks also took substantial time in the Heart Attack–REACT project, which lasted only eighteen months. The project first gained community leaders' support, then greater public awareness, then numerous invitations for public speaking, and finally, in some cities, active interest from the medical community (Heart Attack/REACT Web site, 1999). Moreover, REACT communities continued to penetrate into new social networks and to gain the interest of new groups and associations throughout the project period. Under these circumstances, a different understanding may be needed as to when community programs are ready to be evaluated.

It is not "failings" of community organizations that "cause" these delays; professionals often need time to learn how to work with CBOs. For example, the Pittsburgh collaboration on teenage homicide prevention has exceeded the expected amount of time required for development and implementation. At the university, more time has been necessary than planned to establish procedures and policies permitting the collaboration. In the CBO, building the infrastructure necessary to participate has also taken much longer than anticipated.

Relationships Between Community Capacity Building and Specific Goal Attainment. Once community capacity is identified or developed, what then? There is no reason to believe that increased capacity would have to be addressed to any single health or social problem. Researchers assume that capacity is developed *for* something, but perhaps the intended goal is not the one for which capacity is used. The increased community capacity may help to achieve other goals. Certainly every effort should be made to harness capacity to a specific aim if CBOs received money and made promises. Nevertheless, the positive effects that are seen may not be the ones that were anticipated. Under these circumstances, a discovery capacity may be the only way to document or reveal the actual achievements.

Two examples make the point. The Detroit Halloween Arson Prevention project emerged directly out of community organization efforts throughout the city (Maciak, Moore, Leviton, and Guinan, 1998). The project accessed existing community capacity: any citizen, no matter how impaired, could look outside the door and report on fires being set. It built community capacity by identifying the areas that experienced the most fires and then deployed community volunteers to those locations. However, no data collection effort was ever envisioned. Instead, a discovery process was set in motion after the fact, when the community leaders identified this achievement to CDC staff. Fortunately, fires are reportable, and the volunteer sign-ups were reported by the newspaper. This information permitted the creation of a short time series.

The Pittsburgh Teen Homicide prevention project illustrates that the increase in capacity can either succeed or fail at any given time point and for any specific goal. So far the effort has not appeared to have much effect on the rate of teenage homicide (and it is certainly premature to reach this conclusion). And yet the CBO has seen a blossoming in terms of related activities that are valuable in themselves: increased employment in a low-income neighborhood and increased positive recreation and developmental activities for children. The reduction in homicide will take time and may never be achieved. Perhaps the theory behind the intervention is wrong. Certainly no program, whether professional or community driven, has succeeded very well in reducing teenage homicide. Yet the side effects are very real, and if we uncouple the program assumptions, they cannot be called side effects.

Community Invention and Reinvention. Community-based projects also continue to invent and reinvent strategies to deal with local circumstances in health promotion and disease prevention, even after establishment of an intervention plan. The Community Demonstration Projects of CDC institutionalized such reinvention within an overall strategy. In the Community Demonstration Projects, the basic strategies were consistent from the beginning and were agreed on by the various sites. However, the way in which local sites implemented those strategies had to differ, and they did so by design. For example, the development and dissemination of role model stories to encourage condom use played a large role in the project. However, role model stories were developed locally, a strategy that had great appeal for the community members who were the targets of behavior change. Also, new approaches and new methods to make the stories relevant, attention getting, and persuasive were ongoing throughout the intervention period.

John McKnight (1987, 1995; McKnight and Kretzman, 1990) would understand this creative process very well. McKnight contrasts the way that professionals view the world with the way that community members view the world. Where professionals are hierarchical, formal, and systematic (read "scientific"), communities are spontaneous and creative. Ideas continue to bubble up from community processes as members of associations tackle shared problems. Some of the proposed solutions may not work, but community processes are seldom hampered by a design or intervention protocol. An important role for evaluators, then, is to identify, document, and evaluate the ongoing process of adding to and revising intervention strategies (and also to anticipate which strategies will be unworkable).

Continuing Change Requires Discovery. For many reasons, then, community-based programs have a special need for discovery. Such evaluations are new, the development of the programs and of community capacity takes time, the results may not be those that are expected, and innovation is ongoing in communities to adopt and adapt strategies to the problem at hand. Discovery capacity can assist evaluators in coping with these features and offering valuable insights about community-based programs. In fact, discovery in this context might be defined, in part, as documenting the innovations that take place when community members are exposed to something new and attempt to make meaning of it within their realm of experience.

The Value of Discovery at Different Program Stages

Communities' innovations and their ingenuity in adapting to the circumstances at hand provide important ideas for dissemination and adoption at new locations. Documenting these adaptations yields insights about both program theory and implementation.

Formative Evaluation Stage: Teen Homicide Prevention. Both the AIDS Community Demonstration Projects and the Heart Attack–REACT project had a formal stage of qualitative data gathering from community members. However, the Teen Homicide Prevention project indicates how good results can come from an informal dialogue between professionals and community leaders. In the context of initial program development and piloting, community leaders challenged two key assumptions of the professionals. A psychiatrist with the project brought up the topic of family dysfunction resulting from fatherless households. The CBO's director objected to that characterization, saying that all of these youth had fathers, and most of the fathers lived in the same community. The problem was not how to make up the deficit but how to bridge the distance. A second insight came from a discussion of gang membership and how to encourage youths to quit that life. The director, himself a former gang member, was adamant that he did not want to encourage youths to leave gangs. His view was that the gang was the strongest social support that many youths possessed, and he did not want to take that away from them. Rather, his view was that it would be better if gangs could be redirected so that they were less alienated and could promote greater community safety. Through trial and error, both of these issues are now being addressed.

Two types of information revealed the high risk of reinjury among the youths seen in the emergency department (ED). The director of the trauma service was looking for relief. He told of a youth who had been shot during one of the summer holidays: "I gave up my holiday to save the kid's life." By that winter, he found himself giving up yet another holiday to save the very same kid. He identified this as a pattern: seriously wounded youths entered the ED demanding him for their physician because he had done so well before.

At the same time, one of us (Schuh) maintained an informal database on injury using public sources, the county health department's surveillance unit, and the coroner's records. The database, which records both victim and perpetrator data related to the Homewood neighborhood (the incident occurred in Homewood or one of the actors is a resident of Homewood), is beginning to show names more than once over time: as victim/victim, perpetrator/perpetrator, or victim/perpetrator. By high risk, we mean high risk of being shot again or of shooting someone else (or multimodal injuries such as may be caused by a handgun and baseball bat). By high risk, we mean high risk of being shot again or of shooting someone else (or multimodal injuries such as may be caused by a handgun and baseball bat).

A final insight emerged about adult involvement to obtain consent for the project, and it took a year and a half to document. It emerged that even when adults accompanied the youths to the ED, consent could not be obtained because the adults were supporting the lies (age, circumstances, names, and addresses) that the youths made up on admission. A neighborhood outreach worker discovered the problem when he recognized some youths on the trauma ward who had not been referred to the CBO for follow-up. When he stopped to chat with them, they asked him to be careful to use their aliases while in the hospital. They had provided false names, addresses, and identification. For the database, we tried to compare trauma service names with records from other sources. We discovered that sometimes what appeared to be two individuals turned out to be only one using different names. Even when the parental name and address were available, the parents frequently prevented the CBO from making contact with their sons.

Program Operation Stage: Heart Attack–REACT. This project was implemented in ten communities that varied in their demographics, resources available, and complexity of the medical care system. Data collection mechanisms included abstraction of data from medical charts (an expensive undertaking), a formal protocol to report process information, and three telephone surveys of general community members (concerning awareness of the REACT message), patients released from the hospital after a diagnosis of myocardial infarction, and patients sent home from the ED where myocardial infarction was ruled out. However, several investigators were not satisfied that these data collection strategies would ensure discovery of important insights. Educational campaigns to make people aware of heart attack symptoms and the importance of early action had been studied primarily in Europe, before REACT began. Only two studies had been conducted in the United States. For this reason, there was a great deal of uncertainty about how implementation was actually proceeding; people were literally learning as they went. An improved discovery mechanism was needed, although resources were slender.

One year into the intervention period, and again at the end of intervention (after eighteen months), focus groups of interventionists and their supervisors were conducted by one of us (Leviton) to gain these insights. These were then summarized and provided to all sites for further input and correction. (The findings can be seen in their entirety on the REACT Web site, Heart Attack/REACT, 1997.) The focus groups revealed some unexpected features about REACT that could have gone unnoticed if no one had collected the information systematically. To date, the focus groups have proved at least as useful and informative as the other process-related databases. Moreover, because the other process evaluation efforts were planned in advance with close-ended data collection, they were not capable of providing these insights.

For example, REACT interventionists emphasized a persistent and general point about the message: "It sells itself." People were often squeamish at first about the project ("Yuk! Why would we want to think about heart attacks?"). Other community groups were reluctant to offer support because they worried that the message would frighten people. However, once they understood the basic message ("Save your heart by seeking help early"), the project developed great appeal. Soon REACT staff were invited to all sorts of community events, health fairs, and self-help groups to give their message. This feature was doubly important because it attracted additional community resources. Community leaders and gatekeepers for media developed a positive view of the project and were more willing to provide their own time and resources to the effort.

Furthermore, interventionists learned how flexible and positive the REACT message really was. This was not understood in advance. One interventionist noted that the message was "chameleon-like" in its simplicity. Because it was simple, anyone could give it: people who had experienced heart attack, home health aides in senior high rises, and volunteers in hospital cardiac units. Because the message was positive, it could fit in anywhere: a cardiac rehabilitation group in Texas; golf courses and bingo parlors in Massachusetts; or a senior center potluck supper in Opelika, Alabama.

The discovery data challenged the investigators' assumptions concerning medical care providers. Only after the focus groups did investigators realize that provider interest grew in identifiable stages. Although provider education was intensive from the very start, physicians were slow to respond. By contrast, nurses, paramedics, and other health personnel were key resources throughout the community trial to get the REACT message out to patients and community members. Early in the project, the most one could hope for was endorsement by cardiologists and emergency physicians. Only after the project had been in the field for over a year did other physicians begin to develop a real interest in the message. In Brownsville, Texas, for example, providers did not exhibit much interest at first. By the end of the project, a continuing medical education session had over sixty attendees, and "no one's beeper went off—even once." Variation in this pattern was also noteworthy. In Eau Claire, Wisconsin, physicians were the mainstay of a professional speakers' bureau to give the REACT message.

These examples are important because they shed light on program theory. The overall appeal of the message was not anticipated, and the relatively late interest of many medical providers was contrary to the initial program assumptions. A third insight concerns implementation, and can be shared, replicated, and assessed. In Brownsville, youth volunteers wanted to go door to door in the barrio to talk with residents individually. However, there was a high fear of crime in the neighborhood. To get people to the door, the youth organized a "parade" together with the ambulances, which blew their sirens and flashed their lights. This commotion attracted residents to the doors to see what was going on. The parade created a public, officially sanctioned atmosphere for the door-to-door work by youth, which meant that residents were not afraid to talk to them.

Program Operation Stage: The Partners Continuum of Services. While qualitative methods served discovery in the case of REACT, quantitative program records assisted discovery for the Partners Continuum. A computerized client-tracking management information system (MIS) was implemented in the project and has revealed some important needs for change in services. Schuh and Leviton (1991) have described the uses of this MIS for community-based outreach, follow-up, and client advocacy. The Partners Continuum implemented a version of the tracking system early in its development but did not support the system very well until recently. Having obtained a joint grant, the partners were more interested in the tracking system as a method to monitor progress. One of us (Schuh) is reviewing the files of each agency in the collaborative in turn and has discovered systematic underreporting of the level of effort by agency staff. For example, 95 clients were reported to funders prior to the review; that has increased so far to 164. Agencies tended to underreport because they did not see the distinction between a client of the collaborative and a client of the agency; for example, they would miss a parent who was served by the Housing Authority or a community service agency, when the child was served by the Child Development Center. They also missed cases of serial enrollment (for example, the child in services one month and the mother the next month).

A more spectacular underreporting problem concerned referrals and services provided. For the first reporting period, the continuum reported to the funders 538 referrals for service. So far, the review has found at least 799 such referrals for service. Apparently service providers would document what they saw as the primary need (for example, recovery from substance abuse) but not the ancillary needs (such as treatment for sexually transmitted disease), even as they made referrals for those needs. If this is true generally of collaborative arrangements, then collaboratives may not be giving themselves credit for work done. More critically, the new data gave insights about the range of needs addressed by the collaborative. A certain amount of effort and experience are needed to get people to think about a collaborative when at the same time they are thinking about their own agency's eligibility criteria.

Another insight is qualitative, and illustrates that outside professionals can develop their own expertise about the community, a point sometimes lost in the rhetoric of community participation. The area served by the Partners Continuum of Services includes a large housing project that is slated for demolition. The project has been in existence for some forty-five years. Many of the residents have lived there the whole time, and many families have several generations represented. The Partners Continuum was concerned about the disruption of long-standing social support networks. The director of the health clinic corrected them by observing that these were "survival networks" and not merely social support networks. The obvious truth of that observation was stunning. Disruption of social support networks affects quality-of-life issues. Disruption of survival networks affects life itself.

After the Project Has Ended: Data-Based Puzzles. Several of these projects have given rise to important questions about effects. Two examples make the point. The arson prevention project in Detroit discovered that immediately after a youth curfew was imposed in 1985, the fires that youths were most likely to set (trash fires) declined substantially. The curfew is not enforced during the rest of the year—only during the three-day Halloween period. However, if the curfew is responsible for the rapid decline in these fires, then it may be a powerful way to reduce other youth-related problems in the city. To determine whether it is plausible that the curfew is responsible for the decline, the Urban Research Centers are examining data on the time of day during which fires occurred. (Ability to conduct this analysis will depend on the data's quality.) If trash fires were set at all hours prior to 1985 but were set primarily before 6 P.M. after 1985, then the curfew was probably effective, and it might also work for other purposes.

In retrospect, the discovery capacity is sadly lacking for some of these projects. For example, the AIDS Community Demonstration projects discovered a reduction of sexual risk taking among injection drug users due to intervention, but no statistically significant effect on sharing of injection drug equipment or on use of bleach or alcohol to clean such equipment (CDC AIDS Community Demonstration Projects, 1999). Yet the NIDA demonstration programs had found the opposite to be true: a reduction in drug-related HIV risk but not in sexual risk taking (Coyle, Needle, and Normand, 1998). It is suspected that the effects on drug-related risk were not seen because a new set of guidelines on preventing HIV transmission through injection drug use was released to the public during the project period. Unfortunately, the projects' infrastructure for qualitative data collection had been dismantled in order to provide scarce resources to the program intervention and the quantitative data collection effort. Therefore, the hypothesis could not be checked.

Discovery Is Useful but Neglected. We have offered examples of the usefulness of a discovery capacity at all stages of program development and evaluation. These projects could not have been evaluated usefully without such a capacity—or, at least, their usefulness would have been substantially reduced. Discovery is really a part of the natural process resulting from being introduced to new concepts, technologies, skill, and possibilities. In the light of this conclusion, however, one can ask: Why is discovery a neglected strategy in evaluation of public health programs in general, and of these programs in particular?

Barriers to Maintaining a Capacity for Discovery in Program Evaluation

As these examples indicate, many benefits and insights for programs can result from an ongoing discovery process, especially in community-based programs. However, the examples also illustrate several barriers and typical syndromes that can interfere with maintaining an adequate discovery capacity in program evaluation.

The Preordinate Mind-Set. The priority that is given to summative evaluations often hampers the discovery capacity of programs. Stake (1975, 1978) contrasted responsive evaluation to what he termed "preordinate" evaluation, in which the research question is determined in advance, along with the design and specific measures. In preordinate evaluation, a plan and protocol must be strictly adhered to over time. New discoveries about practice are viewed with suspicion since they can, and often do, change the underlying intervention. Yet discoveries about practice are likely to continue into the summative evaluation, especially in areas where practice is new. In preordinate evaluation, measures must be standardized from the start. Unfortunately, data collection of other kinds is often curtailed severely because people become so focused on the outcome. In preordinate evaluation, the goal of data collection and analysis is set in advance and does not change in the light of new developments in communities or in practice. If these are detected, they are often regarded as nuisance variables, to be controlled in the interest of improved interpretation. On the contrary, they are not nuisance variables; they are sometimes key variables that provide insight concerning why the project does or does not work, how it might be improved, and how it might be replicated.

Let us be clear: we would sometimes prefer to use the experimental method in community settings, because in the final analysis we must test whether an approach is worth the time, money, and effort. Even when the effort is driven by community members, they themselves are entitled to know whether their efforts are worthwhile or whether they should be devoting their hard-won volunteer time to something else. Under the right circumstances, the experimental method can offer the best answer to this question. However, the experimental method has become so deeply ingrained in public health circles that it is sometimes applied when it is not appropriate. One size does not fit all for intervention in communities, at least not yet, for problems for which no one has found an adequate solution.

The case of teenage homicide offers a noteworthy example, because well-intentioned efforts can inhibit discovery. A funder recently held meetings with representatives of several communities as well as experts in the field of violence and victimization. The purpose was to develop a proposal for a demonstration that would include three or four cities. At the initial meeting, it was clear that the communities shared a common concern, but they approached that concern in different ways. One community was employing a faith-based approach working through local clergy and churches. A second city was employing a professional surveillance and monitoring strategy, and a third site was a neighborhood-based response to the problem. The variation in these efforts offered a unique opportunity to explore and compare different locally initiated responses, but it was not explored. Instead of implementing a formative process in each community, the group planned a demonstration with an intervention strategy in common and also common data elements. Some local variation remained, of course. But in general, it was ignored in pilot testing. The opportunity was lost to discover what different types of community capacity could offer to address the problem.

The arson-prevention program offers another example: its serendipity has led to some fairly strange reactions that can be attributed to a preordinate mind-set. Specifically, there have been two critical reactions to this study: that it is not scientific and that it is not a public health program. (One could ask how many charred bodies are required to give it public health significance.) It is important to inquire about the reasons for these statements. In fact, the program simply violated people's expectations. We have become so accustomed to professionally driven interventions, even in community settings, that it becomes difficult to recognize a grassroots intervention when we see it. No public health professional was involved; therefore, it was not public health. Also, we are accustomed to a planned data collection effort, or at least a recognized health surveillance effort; the arson data were not surveillance data as such.

In truth, people were appropriately concerned about the study data. Although the fires were reportable, the Detroit fire department is operating on slender resources for both service delivery and fire investigation. It is not yet clear whether more detailed analysis is justified. In the same way, the counts of volunteer enrollments each Halloween were reported by the newspaper. There is no way to assess the accuracy of the reporting. However, we submit that many professionally driven evaluations keep counts of volunteers in much the same way and never bring them under close scrutiny. Implementation data are seldom assessed for validity.

Allocation of Scarce Resources. The quality of the arson data, like the underreporting of services in the Partners Continuum, points to a problem: community programs may have little experience in data collection and limited budgets for it. These obstacles can certainly harm evaluations and lead to more negative conclusions than may be warranted. In addition, the discovery capacity can suffer even in well-funded studies. The reason is that program implementation and outcome evaluation absorb so much of the study's budget. For example, the primary outcome of the Heart Attack–REACT evaluation required abstracting thousands of medical records, an enormously expensive data collection effort. As a result, ancillary data collection efforts, such as surveys of community awareness, were left with minimal resources. In the same way, the AIDS Community Demonstration projects could no longer justify maintaining an extensive infrastructure for qualitative data once the formative research stage was complete. Yet much might have been learned about implementation and about changes in the communities if more qualitative data collection had been permitted to continue.

Overcoming the Focus on "Doing." The REACT study reinforced an important principle concerning discovery. Program staff, and often the researchers themselves, became fully engaged in "doing" because the program was time limited, and much had to be accomplished in order to achieve the goal. It becomes difficult under these circumstances to get people to engage in introspection. To allow introspection, it was necessary to take Heart Attack–REACT staff out of their daily context, through a retreat that offered the opportunity for focus groups. An alternative would be to include a qualitative observer or participant observer in all program activities. However, the cost was prohibitive for ten widely scattered intervention communities, given the resources available, the priority assigned to medical chart abstraction, and the likely payoff.

Overcoming Accountability Mind-Set in Process Evaluation. Program staff are prone to focus on accountability or reporting requirements as the most important purpose of process evaluation. This emphasis is often reinforced by supervisors. For example, initially the REACT investigators requested that intervention staff submit monthly narratives about what they were discovering in the field: opportunities, obstacles, and facilitators to get the message out. Regardless of instructions, what the investigators received was a narrative report on performance accountability (for example, "We participated in ten community meetings this month"). The focus on accountability can interfere substantially with ongoing staff cooperation in discovery. For one thing, rewards and punishments flow from such reporting requirements; staff want to be seen as "doing a good job" and may assume that reporting assesses their performance, whether it does so or not. A discovery focus tries to break this mind-set, at least briefly, by asking them to reflect on what is actually going on in the program.

Conclusion

Ample evidence suggests the special importance of a discovery capacity for programs that are community based and community driven. This discovery can be important to inform the theory underlying a program approach and to understand implementation better. Because communities are innovative while evaluation is selective, discovery in evaluation can operate to select the best of community creation. However, it is not always possible to anticipate where the successes will be. Community-based efforts often labor under conditions of lower resources, less respect from professionals, and the need to prove themselves capable. A discovery capacity in evaluation is suited to addressing these problems.

The Heart Attack/REACT program was funded by grants from the National Heart, Lung and Blood Institute, National Institutes of Health, Bethesda, Maryland (U01 HL 53142; 54517; 53211; 53135; 53141; and 53149). The Pilot Project to Provide Mental Health and Community-based Services to Adolescent and Youth Victims of Violence from Homewood is supported by a grant from the Stanton Farm Foundation. The Partners Continuum of Services is supported, in part, by grants from the R. K. Mellon Foundation and a grant from the U.S. Department of Housing and Urban Development. Laura Leviton's participation in the Detroit Arson Prevention evaluation was made possible through an interagency personnel arrangement with the Urban Research Centers, Epidemiology Program Office, Centers for Disease Control and Prevention. Information concerning the AIDS Community Demonstration Projects was provided by personal communications with Donna Higgins, the acting director of the CDC Urban Research Centers.

References

Alinsky, S. D. *Rules for Radicals: A Practical Primer for Realistic Radicals.* New York: Vintage Books, 1972.

CDC AIDS Community Demonstration Projects Research Group. "The CDC AIDS Community Demonstration Projects: A Multi-site Community-level Intervention to Promote HIV Risk Reduction." *American Journal of Public Health,* 1999, 89, 336–345.

Clark, N. M., and McLeroy, K. R. "Creating Capacity Through Health Education: What We Know and What We Don't." *Health Education Quarterly,* 1995, 22, 273–289.

"Community-Level Prevention of Human Immunodeficiency Virus Infection Among High-Risk Populations: The AIDS Community Demonstration Projects." *Morbidity and Mortality Weekly Report,* May 10, 1996, pp. 1–24.

Cornell, C. E., for the Uniontown Community Health Project Group. "SIP 18W: Peer Support Intervention for CVD Risk Reduction in African-American Women, Aged 40 and Older: Progress Report and Update." Paper presented at the Ninth Annual Prevention Research Centers Conference, Atlanta, Feb. 2, 1999.

Coyle, S. L., Needle, R. H., and Normand, J. "Outreach-based HIV Prevention for Injecting Drug Users: A Review of Published Outcome Data." *Public Health Reports,* 1998, 113, Suppl. 1, 19–30.

Eng, E., Parker, E., and Harlan, C. "Lay Health Advisor Intervention Strategies: A Continuum from Natural Helping to Paraprofessional Helping." *Health Education and Behavior,* 1997, 24, 413–417.

Etzioni, A. *The Spirit of Community.* New York: Crown, 1993.

Finnegan, J. R., and others. "Delay in Seeking Care for Heart Attack Symptoms: Findings from National Focus Groups." *Health Communication,* forthcoming.

Freire, P. *Pedagogy of the Oppressed.* New York: Herder and Herder, 1970.

Green, L. W., and Kreuter, M. W. *Health Promotion Planning: An Educational and Environmental Approach.* (2nd ed.) Mountain View, Calif.: Mayfield, 1991.

Guenther-Grey, C., Noroian, D., Fonseka, J., and Higgins, D. "Developing Community Networks to Deliver HIV Prevention Interventions." *Public Health Reports,* 1996, 111, Suppl. 1, 41–49.

Heart Attack/REACT Web Site. "Notes from the Field," 1997. http://www.epi.umn.edu/react. Division of Epidemiology, School of Public Health, University of Minnesota.

Higgins, D. L., and others. "Using Formative Research to Lay the Foundation for Community Level HIV Prevention Efforts: An Example from the AIDS Community Demonstration Projects." *Public Health Reports,* 1996, 111, Suppl. 1, 28–35.

Leviton, L. C. "Program Theory and Evaluation Theory in Community-based Programs." *Evaluation Practice,* 1994, 15, 89–92.

Leviton, L. C., Needleman, C. E., and Shapiro, M. *Confronting Public Health Risks: A Decision Maker's Guide.* Thousand Oaks, Calif.: Sage, 1998.

Leviton, L. C., and Schuh, R. G. "Evaluation of Outreach as a Program Element." *Evaluation Review,* 1990, 15, 420–440.

Leviton, L. C., and others. "Formative Research Methods to Understand Patient and Provider Responses to Heart Attack Symptoms." *Evaluation and Program Planning,* forthcoming.

Lipsey, M. W. "Practice and Malpractice in Evaluation Research." *Evaluation Practice,* 1988, 9, 5–25.

Lipsey, M. W. *Design Sensitivity: Statistical Power for Experimental Research.* Thousand Oaks, Calif.: Sage, 1990.

Lipsey, M. W., and others. "Evaluation: The State of the Art and the Sorry State of the Science." In D. Cordray (ed.), *Utilizing Prior Research in Evaluation Planning.* New Directions for Program Evaluation, no. 27. San Francisco: Jossey-Bass, 1985.

Maciak, B., Moore, M., Leviton, L. C., and Guinan, M. "Preventing Halloween Arson in an Urban Setting." *Health Education and Behavior,* 1998, 25, 194–211.

McAlister, A. L. "Population Behavior Change: A Theory-Based Approach." *Journal of Public Health Policy,* 1991, *12,* 345–361.

McKnight, J. L. "Regenerating Community." *Social Policy,* 1987, *17,* 54–58.

McKnight, J. L. *The Careless Society: Community and Its Counterfeits.* New York: Basic Books, 1995.

McKnight, J. L., and Kretzmann, J. P. *Mapping Community Capacity.* Evanston, Ill.: Center for Urban Affairs and Policy Research, Northwestern University, 1990.

Reichardt, C. S. "Summative Evaluation, Formative Evaluation, and Tactical Research." *Evaluation Practice,* 1994, *15,* 275–281.

Rogers, E. M. *Diffusion of Innovations.* New York: Free Press, 1983.

Schuh, R. G., and Leviton, L. C. "Evaluating Referral and Agency Coordination with a Computerized Client Tracking System." *Evaluation Review,* 1991, *15,* 533–554.

Schuh, R. G., Marin, R., Thompson, K., and Byrdsong, R. "Prevention of Injury from Youth Violence: Role of Formative Evaluation in Developing Demonstration Programs." Paper presented at the American Evaluation Association Annual Meeting, San Diego, Calif., Nov. 1997.

Scriven, M. "The Methodology of Evaluation." In R. W. Tyler, R. M. Gagne, and M. Scriven (eds.), *Perspectives of Curriculum Evaluation.* Skokie, Ill.: Rand McNally, 1967.

Simon, H. A. *The Sciences of the Artificial.* Cambridge, Mass.: MIT Press, 1970.

Simons, P. Z., and others. "Building a Peer Network for a Community Level HIV Prevention Program Among Injecting Drug Users in Denver." *Public Health Reports,* 1996, *111,* Suppl. 1, 50–153.

Simons-Morton, D. G., and others. "Rapid Early Action for Coronary Treatment (REACT): Rationale, Design, and Baseline Characteristics." Submitted to *Academic Emergency Medicine,* 1999.

Stake, R. E. (ed.). *Evaluating the Arts in Education: A Responsive Approach.* Columbus, Ohio: Merrill, 1975.

Stake, R. E. "The Case Study Method in Social Inquiry." *Educational Researcher,* 1978, *7,* 5–8.

Suchman, E. A. "Action for What? A Critique of Evaluative Research." In R. O'Toole (ed.), *The Organization, Management and Tactics of Social Research.* Cambridge, Mass.: Schenkman Publishing Co., 1970.

Weiss, C. *Evaluation* (2nd ed.) Englewood Cliffs, N.J.: Prentice Hall, 1998.

Wholey, J. S. "Evaluability Assessment: Developing Program Theory." In L. Bickman (ed.), *Using Program Theory in Evaluation.* New Directions for Program Evaluation, no. 33. San Francisco: Jossey-Bass, 1987.

Wholey, J. S. "Assessing the Feasibility and Likely Usefulness of Evaluation." In J. S. Wholey, H. P. Hatry, and K. E. Newcomer (eds.), *Handbook of Practical Program Evaluation.* San Francisco: Jossey-Bass, 1994.

Zapka, J., Estabrook, B., Gilliland, J., Leviton, L., and others. "Health Care Providers' Perspectives on Patient Delay for AMI Symptom Care-Seeking." *Journal of Health Behavior and Health Education,* forthcoming.

Laura C. Leviton was professor in the Department of Health Behavior, School of Public Health, University of Alabama at Birmingham and is now senior program officer for research and evaluation at the Robert Wood Johnson Foundation.

Russell G. Schuh is internal evaluator for a community-based, grassroots violence prevention program, as well as evaluator of agency-based programs for community outreach programs and welfare-to-work programs in Pittsburgh.

Central to most community-based programs is the goal of improving the community's capacity to address its own problems. Evaluating changes in community capacity requires contextualized definitions that (1) respect geographic, political, academic, and community perspectives and (2) inclusive evaluation approaches.

Evaluating Community-Based Health Programs That Seek to Increase Community Capacity

Edith A. Parker, Eugenia Eng, Amy J. Schulz, Barbara A. Israel

Critical reflection and new opportunities for funding in the field of public health have given rise to a number of partnership approaches to research and practice (Israel, Schulz, Parker, and Becker, 1998). These approaches, often referred to as community based, have called for increased attention to the complex issues that compromise the health of people living in marginalized communities; more integration of research and practice; greater community involvement and control; increased sensitivity to and competence in working within diverse cultures; expanded use of both qualitative and quantitative research methods; and more focus on health and quality of life (Israel, Schulz, Parker, and Becker, 1998).

A central tenet of this emphasis on community-based public health research and practice is the importance of building on and enhancing the strengths and problem-solving capacity of communities as an objective of interventions aimed at promoting health and preventing disease. This recognition of the importance of community capacity for health promotion has a long tradition in public health, with explication in the 1940s by South Africans Steuart and his colleagues Kark and Cassell (Trostle, 1986). In Steuart's social change model, increasing community problem-solving capacity to address barriers to good health is an objective that is as important as improving health status itself (Eng, Salmon, and Mullan, 1992; Steckler, Dawson, Israel, and Eng, 1993; Steuart, 1993; Trostle, 1986). Despite recognition of the role of community capacity in health promotion, few attempts to evaluate changes in community capacity have been reported in the literature.

This chapter describes key issues to consider in evaluating community capacity based on four community-based health programs that have included increasing community capacity or a related concept as one of the defined objectives of their program and their subsequent evaluations. Two are programs in rural areas, and the other two are in large urban settings. Three of the four programs target general health, and the fourth program focuses on improving the health of women and children.

Definitions of Community Capacity

Despite recognition of the relationship of community capacity to health promotion, there is no clear consensus on the operational definition of *community capacity*. For example, *community capacity* is often used interchangeably with other, similar concepts such as *community competence* (Cottrell, 1976; Eng and Parker, 1994; Goeppinger and Baglioni, 1985), *sense of community* (McMillan and Chavis, 1986), and *empowerment* (Israel, Checkoway, Schulz, and Zimmerman, 1994; Wallerstein, 1992). Yet all three of these concepts differ from each other. A *competent community* is defined as one in which the various parts of the community are able to collaborate effectively in identifying the problems and needs of the community, can achieve a working consensus on goals and priorities, can agree on ways and means to implement the agreed-on goal, and can collaborate effectively in the required actions (Cottrell, 1976). *Sense of community* is defined as opportunities in a community for membership, influence, mutual needs to be met, and shared emotional ties and support. An *empowered community* is one in which individuals and organizations collectively use their skills and resources to meet their respective needs. Within an empowered community, there are opportunities for citizen participation in decision making and interaction between individuals and organizations. Through this participation and interaction, individuals and organizations support each other, address conflicts within the community, and gain influence and control over the quality of life in their community. An empowered community has the ability to influence decisions and changes in the larger social system (Israel, Checkoway, Schulz, and Zimmerman, 1994).

Given this lack of consensus on the definition of community capacity, the Division of Chronic Disease Control and Community Intervention, Centers for Disease Control and Prevention (CDC), convened a two-day symposium in 1995 as a process for further specifying and clarifying the dimensions that are integral to community capacity (Goodman and others, 1998). The participants represented a wide range of disciplines, including community health development, health education, community psychology, epidemiology, anthropology, political science, and sociology. At the symposium, participants engaged in a series of facilitated discussions around the definition of community capacity, and dimensions of community capacity were identified. Participants were then assigned to work groups that corresponded to each dimension. Over the next few months, the work groups researched these dimensions, and their findings were synthesized in an article describing and analyzing the dimensions of community capacity. The dimensions delineated are citizen participation and leadership, skills, resources, social and interorganizational networks, sense of community, understanding of community history, community power, community values, and critical reflection (Goodman and others, 1998).

This definition encompasses many of the constructs others have used in evaluating community capacity and related phenomena. For example, elements of community empowerment can be found in the dimensions of power, values, and critical reflection. In addition, sense of community is listed as a dimension of community capacity (as opposed to its previous conceptualization as a separate but related concept to community capacity). Components of community competence are also included in the dimensions of participation and leadership, skills, and social and interorganizational networks.

This framework for community capacity highlights the challenge for evaluators in seeking a single definition and operationalization of community capacity building. As Goodman and colleagues noted, the dimensions of community capacity in their framework are broad but not exhaustive, and capacity is a construct that has different meanings in different contexts. Some evaluators have suggested that the context of communities is so unique that one operational definition of community capacity is not possible (Eng and Parker, 1994). Others suggest that concepts such as community competence and community empowerment are not dimensions or aspects of community capacity (as suggested in the framework) but very different concepts, which relate directly to the goals of the program or the context of the community in which the program is implemented.

In short, the definition and operationalization of community capacity are still evolving. The purpose of this chapter is not to resolve these defined issues but rather to present examples of community-based health programs that have assessed different dimensions of community capacity and to identify common key lessons learned from each of these evaluation experiences. Each of the case studies described here used a slightly different operationalization of community capacity in evaluating program process, impact, and outcomes.

Case Examples of Evaluations of Programs Seeking to Enhance Community Capacity

The following section describes the four community health projects and their evaluations that serve as case studies for this chapter.

East Side Village Health Worker Partnership. This is a project of the Detroit Community Academic Urban Research Center, funded by the CDC. Its broad goal is to improve the health of women and children in the targeted area within east side Detroit through the involvement of lay health advisers, referred to as village health workers (VHWs) in this project (Parker, Schulz, Israel, and

Hollis, 1998). A participatory action research approach is being used to ensure that the lay health adviser model is adapted to the context and setting of this particular urban area. The partnership involves an extensive evaluation research component that uses a single case study design and a combination of quantitative and qualitative data collection methods, including participant observations and field notes of steering committee meetings, VHW training, monthly meetings of VHWs and special events; a seven-hundred-household face-to-face random sample community survey conducted in the first and fifth years of the project; pre-and posttraining assessment of VHWs; focus group interviews with VHWs; in-depth interviews with VHWs, steering committee members, community key informants, health department staff, and agency and community-based organization staff; and documentation records by VHWs and staff.

Aspects of community capacity assessed through the evaluation of the VHW partnership include opportunity for participation, skills and resources available to community members and lay health advisers involved with the project; social and interorganizational networks; sense of community; commitment to community; perceptions of organizational and community influence; and perceptions of shared values. To operationalize these aspects of community capacity in the household survey, evaluators have included measures of a sense of community (McMillan and Chavis, 1986), empowerment (Israel, Checkoway, Schulz, and Zimmerman's perceived control scale, 1994), community competence (items from Eng and Parker's community competence scale, 1994, with items developed based on the work of Warren and Warren, 1977), and social integration and informal social control (measured with a four-item social integration scale and a four-item informal social control scale) (Sampson, Raudenbush, and Earls, 1997). In addition, respondents in the qualitative in-depth interviews are asked about their perceptions of the problem-solving capacity of their neighborhoods.

Partners for Improved Nutrition and Health (PINAH). This program was implemented in 1988 as a five-year collaborative effort by the Freedom from Hunger Foundation, the Mississippi State Department of Health, and the Mississippi Cooperative Extension Agency. The project targeted communities in three small towns in a county in the Mississippi delta. The three overall goals were to improve the health-seeking behaviors of community residents, enhance the problem-solving capacity of local relational communities, and improve outreach and referral patterns of local health and human service agencies. To achieve these goals, PINAH staff recruited and trained lay health advisers from the three communities in basic health information, counseling, and community organization techniques (Eng and Parker, 1994).

The PINAH project also employed a participatory action research approach to evaluation. Four structured data collection instruments were developed to collect quantitative data to assess community competence, interagency referrals, and two separate instruments on community health advisers' (CHA) helping activities with the members of their social networks. Qualitative data collection methods included individual in-depth and focus group interviews with community health advisers and service providers, parents, teenagers, senior citizens, people helped by the lay health advisers, interagency council members, community residents, respondents to the annual quantitative community competence survey, and PINAH staff.

To assess community competence, PINAH evaluators used Cottrell's community competence construct as a starting point to develop, with community member input, a closed-ended questionnaire. This instrument included items intending to measure Cottrell's eight dimensions of community competence (participation, articulateness, communication, self-other awareness, management of relations with larger society, machinery for facilitating participant interaction, conflict containment and accommodation, and commitment) as well as the added dimension of social support. Qualitative interviews also included questions about perceived changes in these dimensions of community competence.

In 1992, the W. K. Kellogg Foundation launched the four-year, $16 million Community-Based Public Health Initiative (CBPH) in response to suggestions outlined in the 1988 Institute of Medicine's *Report on the Future of Public Health* and to concerns about the growing disparity in health status between the have and have-not communities. The CBPH initiative was designed to strengthen linkages between public health education and public health practice by forming formal partnerships among academia, health agencies, and people in communities. To be eligible for the program, each site had to form a consortium consisting of a school or an academic program of public health, at least one other health professions school, one or more communities with serious public health problems, and the local public health agencies of these communities. North Carolina and Michigan were two of the seven national sites funded through this initiative (Brownson, Riley, and Bruce, 1998).

North Carolina Community-Based Public Health Initiative (NC CBPHI). The NC CBPHI consists of four separate county coalitions, each of which is focusing project activities within a community in that county (Parker and others, 1998; Eng and others, 1999). Members of each of the coalitions include, at the minimum, representatives from the University of North Carolina Schools of Public Health and Medicine, the health department of that county, at least one community-based organization, one primary health care center, and representatives from the community with which the coalition is working. Although the specific objectives of each of the four county coalitions differ slightly in wording and in indicators, the coalitions share common objectives:

To increase the problem-solving capacity of the relational community with which the coalition is working

To improve the health status of minority and high-risk populations in selected communities

To increase the ability of agencies within that county to work with the communities they serve to bring about change

To establish an interorganizational network that will increase collaboration among community service agencies, the university, and community members to serve better the minority or high-risk populations in the communities with which the coalition is working

To improve the skills of School of Public Health faculty and students to work with minority and high-risk populations

To recruit minority youth from the participating county into health-related careers (Eng and others, 1999)

Evaluation of the NC CBPHI employed a multiple case study participatory evaluation design with each county coalition, the overall consortium, and academic partners serving as single cases. Evaluation reports for each of these cases were generated at baseline, Year 2, Year 3, and Year 4 of the project (the final funded year from the Kellogg Foundation). Data sources for these reports included annual in-depth qualitative interviews with coalition members (an average of forty interviews per year for the four coalitions), participant observations of coalition meetings and sponsored events (an average of sixty events across the four coalitions each year), a review of coalition documents, and a health agency survey and survey of School of Public Health faculty that were administered in Years 2 and 4 of the project.

To assess changes in community capacity, the NC CBPHI evaluation focused primarily on changes in the ability of the community partners to participate as full partners in all coalition decisions and activities and to be recognized as equal partners by agency and university coalition partners. For example, the evaluation sought to measure the extent to which community partners were not only at the table but played a key role in driving the goals, objectives, and activities of the coalitions. The evaluation also sought to measure changes in community competence in the communities that were the focus of coalition activities. Qualitative in-depth interviews and focus groups were primarily used to evaluate changes in these aspects of community capacity and community competence. Questions for the interview guides in these interviews were developed based on criteria and indicators jointly developed by the coalition members.

Broome Team of Genesee County, Michigan Community-Based Public Health. The Community-Based Public Health Initiative in Michigan focused activities in Detroit and Flint, Michigan, and was called the Detroit-Genesee County Community-Based Public Health Consortium. The partners in Flint named themselves the Broome Team, in honor of a community leader who had been involved in the early planning of the CBPH initiative in Flint. Here we focus on the evaluation activities of the Broome Team.

Broome Team partners included representatives from the University of Michigan School of Public Health and the Health Professions and Studies School at the University of Michigan, Flint; the Genesee County Health Department; and the following community-based organizations: Flint Odyssey House,

Genesee Area Skill Center, Genesee County Community Action Agency, Flint Area Community Economic Development, and Flint Neighborhood Coalition. The two main goals of the Broome Team were to strengthen public health education and practice by linking academic and agency professionals with people from vulnerable neighborhoods and to promote the public's health by enhancing the capacity of community members and community-based organizations. Broome Team used the following evaluation methods:

- Closed-ended questionnaires focusing on the process of the Broome Team meetings
- Monthly reporting forms completed by each of the organizations involved in the Broome Team to document their activities
- A survey of health center staff members conducted in October 1994
- Focus groups conducted with community members who worked with four of the six community based organizations (CBOs) involved with the Broome Team
- Field notes taken at the monthly Broome Team meetings
- In-depth interviews with Broome Team members in Years 1 and 4 of the project
- Follow-up conversations with members of the Broome Team regarding their activities and the relevance of those activities to the goals and objectives of the Broome Team as a whole

In addition, evaluation activities focusing on the School of Public Health, a major partner in the Broome Team, consisted of a faculty survey, field notes at meetings of the community-based public health committee within the school, focus groups with students, a student survey, and in-depth interviews with faculty and students who participated in CBPH activities.

Within the Broome Team, the dimensions of community capacity that were included in the evaluation were citizen participation and leadership; group process (including processes for decision making, resolving differences of opinion, and building trust); participant interaction; decision-making autonomy of organizational representatives to the Broome Team; history with the collaborative group; and perceptions of influences at the individual and organizational levels. These dimensions include aspects of Cottrell's eight dimensions of community competence (Cottrell, 1976), Israel and colleagues' community empowerment (Israel, Checkoway, Schulz, and Zimmerman, 1994), as well as issues identified within the group itself as important aspects of community capacity. Results from the evaluation efforts were used as process indicators within the group and served as discussion tools for members of the Broome Team to examine and address issues related to their collaborative efforts. Over time, these evaluation tools documented evolutions in trust among group members, differences in history with the group (for example, which organizations were able to sustain ongoing involvement with the collaborative and which had less sustained or consistent representation), and differences in perceived decision-making influence within the collaborative body.

Key Issues to Consider in Evaluating Community Capacity

The key issues we present are based on our experience with the evaluations of the four community-based health projects just described. Although these principles and methods are presented as distinct items, they are interrelated, and the order in which they are presented is not meant to suggest a ranking of their importance. Finally, we discuss these issues within the context of advocating for the use of multiple types of evaluation activities (process, impact, outcome, and context) when evaluating health promotion programs seeking to enhance community capacity (Israel and others, 1995).

•*Evaluation of community capacity should use a broad definition of community that includes political and power considerations as well as the geographic boundaries and relationships of the community.* A crucial question facing evaluators of programs attempting to increase community capacity is defining the community. Definitions of community can focus on one or all of the following: geographic elements (an aggregate of individuals residing in a particular place), relational elements (the functions of ties among organizations, neighborhoods, families, and friends), or political elements (the coming together of people to set a political dynamic in motion to transform and act on issues they face) (Heller, 1989; Israel, Checkoway, Schulz, and Zimmerman, 1994; Labonte, 1989; McKnight, 1991). Often programs focus on the first definition of community without considering the second two definitions. Yet consideration of all three of these elements of community can improve understanding of the key factors to focus on in seeking to increase community capacity and evaluate those increases.

Recognition of the political dynamics of a community is especially crucial in community interventions in socially and economically marginalized communities. In operationalizing community capacity, consideration of the political dynamics of that community and how these dynamics affect the health and well-being of those persons involved in the intervention may be particularly useful in identifying the targets of change that the program activities will focus on. For example, in work done with rural communities in Mississippi and North Carolina through the PINAH and CBPHI projects, community residents identified the quality of and access to services as well as access to community facilities as key facilitating factors in enhancing a community's capacity (Parker and Eng, 1995). These residents saw both the quality of services offered and the limited access to services and facilities as grounded in a lack of political clout among these community members and fear of racial integration by the political office-holders in these communities. The PINAH evaluation thus included changes in community service delivery agencies and institutions as part of the desired project outcome of enhanced community competence. To explore these desired changes, qualitative interviews included questions about client satisfaction, access to care, and perceived organizational change in health and social service agencies and questions about changes in the relationships between community members and the power holders within these institutions, agencies, and local government. These questions sought to document changes in the political relationships within the community. Qualitative evaluation data suggested that the community health advisers of the PINAH program had contributed to improvements in service accessibility in two of the intervention communities and increased service availability, quality of services, and service utilization in the third intervention community. In addition, these data suggest that relationships between the community members and agency personnel were improved through the work of the community health advisers (CHAs). Respondents attributed the improvement in the quality of services as a result of feedback to agencies from the CHAs about client satisfaction as well as the extent to which community needs were met. In addition, the CHAs described increases in their ability to make changes in the agencies and institutions in their communities and cited examples where their actions had resulted in improved changes in service agencies.

In addition to influencing relationships between community institutions and communities with which they are working, political dynamics may also affect an evaluator's relationships with community members (Israel, Schulz, Parker, and Becker, 1998). Often socially and economically marginalized communities have not had the power to name or define their own experience in past research and evaluation activities. Recognition and acknowledgment of the inequalities between the evaluator and community participants and how these inequalities among community members may shape their participation and influence in program and evaluation activities will be useful for the evaluator in soliciting participation from community members (Israel, Schulz, Parker, and Becker, 1998). By including political dynamics in the definition of community, the evaluator is able to examine the extent to which influence is shared among health professionals and community members in defining solutions to community health concerns (Eng and Parker, 1994).

In considering the various definitions of a community in health program planning and evaluation, Steuart's conceptualization of units of identity and solution can be extremely useful. In Steuart's schema (1993), there are units of identity (units with which individuals feel themselves to be associated, such as relational communities) and units of solution (defined as units appropriate or essential for the solution of particular problems). Communities of identity may be centered on a defined geographic neighborhood or a geographically dispersed ethnic group with a sense of common identity and shared fate (Israel, Schulz, Parker, and Becker, 1998). For example, neighborhoods may be units of identity if the residents feel a sense of connection and belonging with each other, share needs and aspirations, and experience similar conditions. In any geographically defined city or county, there are likely to be many units of identity. These units of identity are potential units of solution if the members work together in collective problem solving. In addition, for the purposes of community problem solving, different units of identity may need to come together to form units of solution: that is, many units of identity may need to come together, pooling resources to forge a common solution to a problem or concern that they all share. For evaluators of community-based health programs seeking to increase community problem-solving capacity, this distinction means consideration of a community as more than a geographical entity. Identifying the units of identity of the community members involved in an intervention can allow the evaluator to track how these units of identity become units of solution and what partnerships have been formed among the various units of identity to become units of solution.

An example of consideration of both the relational elements and the political dynamics of a community in assessing units of identify and solution can be found in the East Side Village Health Worker Partnership. In this project, extensive consideration has been given to the historical and political context as well as the internal organization of the intervention area. Evaluators noted both strengths and challenges of the intervention area tied to historical events and political context (Parker, Schulz, Israel, and Hollis, 1998). For example, Detroit has traditionally had a large number of single-family households (which could serve as a base for a neighborhood organizing strategy), a history of union and neighborhood organizing, and relatively positive relationships between police and community residents on the east side since the 1970s. Yet Detroit also experiences challenges facing other urban areas, such as past racial tensions and out-migration of population and businesses. Consideration of these broad historical and political factors allowed the evaluators to understand the history and context within which the intervention developed and to examine the evaluation results, including changes in community capacity, in the light of these historical factors.

In addition, to ascertain how a carved-out geographical intervention area corresponded to the internal organization of the area, evaluation staff sought input from the Partnerships' Steering Committee (comprising community-based organization and agency representatives) and also conducted key informant interviews with community members. In these interviews, respondents were asked about their conceptualizations and perceived boundaries of their community, functions of their community, strengths and problems of their community, helping patterns, and history of communal activities. The results of these interviews indicated that residents described their neighborhoods as units of identity, spoke of strong neighborhood-based relationships, and described active block clubs, agency services, churches, and individuals. Respondents also identified neighborhood concerns such as drug dealers, lack of parenting skills, lack of supervised activities for children and youth, and violence.

From this information, evaluators, working with program participants, were able to identify existing units of identity and potential units of solution within the intervention area from which the program could build on in trying to strengthen community capacity. In addition, they were able to identify limits of the evaluation design, which focused on a geographic community with an imperfect match with communities of identity and solution. In doing so, the evaluators and community partners can examine the implications of these differences for the evaluation and intervention design, and discuss potential actions to strengthen the ability of the evaluation to document changes brought about through the intervention.

• *Evaluators working in community settings should define community capacity through the blending of academic and community conceptualizations.* Although there is no clear consensus on the conceptual or operational definition of community capacity, there are several similar constructs to community capacity, such as community competence (Cottrell, 1976; Eng and Parker, 1994), sense of community (McMillan and Chavis, 1986), and community empowerment (Wallerstein, 1992; Israel, Checkoway, Schulz, and Zimmerman, 1994). Each of the case examples in this chapter has used elements of these constructs in the operating definition of community capacity. In addition, to include consideration of the context of the community in which the program is operating, evaluators in each of these examples sought input from community members in confirming (and, if necessary, refining) their definitions of community capacity based on these constructs. Two examples of ways to engage the community in creating a context-specific definition of community capacity can be found in the PINAH project and the East Side Village Health Worker Partnership.

For the PINAH project, evaluators used Cottrell's framework on community competence as the basis to operationalize community capacity. To ensure a directly relevant definition of community competence, PINAH staff conducted two separate half-day workshops with two different community groups. The first group was the local Interagency Council, with representatives from all health and human service agencies in the county. The second group was a local community-based organization of African American leaders that emerged during the civil rights movement. In both workshops, PINAH staff led participants through a structured group exercise to arrive at a consensus on the characteristics they would look for to decide if a community "can get it together" (participants' term to describe community competence). The two groups generated twenty-three traits of a community that "could get it together." Staff then compared these twenty-three traits against Cottrell's eight dimensions of community competence, clustering those that corresponded to one of the dimensions and creating new dimensions from the remaining characteristics. The conclusion was that the twenty-three traits represented four dimensions of community competence—only three of Cottrell's eight dimensions and an additional dimension of social support. Because evaluation staff had no empirical basis for eliminating any of the dimensions (the five dimensions from the literature that were not mentioned by the service providers and community leaders and the new dimension of social support that was contributed by them), the evaluation took the more conservative decision of including all nine dimensions in the development of the community competence questionnaire (Eng and Parker, 1994). This questionnaire was then administered to key informants in each of the three communities.

Results of the baseline and three subsequent years of questionnaire administration supported Cottrell's assertion that community competence is a multidimensional construct. For example, although one of the three communities showed overall gains in the dimensions of participation, social support, commitment, and management of relations with the wider society, it saw no change in conflict containment and accommodation, articulateness, and self-other awareness. Results of the questionnaire administration also raised questions for the evaluators about the ability to capture community competence in a close-ended questionnaire accurately. From the qualitative interview data collected, the evaluation staff learned much about the context of the communities in which community competence was being measured. For example, in the qualitative data, many respondents spoke about racial conflict in some of the communities and how racism affected these communities' ability to solve problems around health and social issues. Because of the closed-ended nature of the questions asked on the questionnaire, none of these key findings arose in the questionnaire data.

In the East Side Village Health Worker Project, project staff developed an initial conceptual framework based on the stress literature of Israel and her colleagues (Israel, Checkoway, Schulz, and Zimmerman, 1994; House, 1981; Katz and Kahn, 1978). This framework postulates that stressors in an individual's environment contribute to an increase in perceived stress in the individual. This increase in perceived stress can then result in short-term responses to stress and strains that may contribute to enduring adverse health outcomes. In this case, the focus was on stressors that affected the health of women and children. Of importance in this conceptual model is the role of conditioning variables: individual and situational characteristics that can affect the process through which stressors are experienced as stressful and can affect the relationship of stressors to health outcomes. Conditioning variables can have a direct relationship to health status, a positive impact on health by buffering the effect of stress, a negative impact by amplifying its effect, or a neutral role. Among the conditioning variables in this conceptual framework of relevance to this discussion are community capacity, community empowerment, social support, accessible services, and existing local, state, and national policies.

To elaborate this framework for the context of the intervention area, project staff sought the input of the steering committee in identifying stressors and conditioning variables present in the East Side. University partners facilitated a group exercise with the steering committee in which members were asked to identify sources of stress for women who care for children on the East Side (stressors), how people feel and respond to these sources of stress (short-term responses to stress), what occurs if these stressors continue over a long time period (enduring health outcomes), and what the factors are that can keep these stressors from having a negative effect on people's lives (conditioning variables). The steering committee generated a list of forty-nine stressors and twenty-five conditioning variables (Schulz and others, 1998). This information was then used as a basis for developing a 350-item survey questionnaire. When conditioning variables identified by the steering committee members were similar to those identified in the literature (for example, sense of community, sense of control, neighbors helping neighbors), evaluation staff used already-existing items from these constructs. For the conditioning variables and stressors identified by the steering committee members with no similar constructs in the literature, evaluation staff developed new questionnaire items. Thus, evaluation staff blended knowledge from the literature with knowledge of community members to create a measurement tool that captures the context of East Side Detroit.

• *Evaluators should use evaluation approaches that enhance community capacity.* Evaluation methods for a program intending to increase community capacity should not contradict or interfere with the goals and values of the stated purpose (Eng and Parker, 1994). The choice of methods and process should facilitate the reciprocal transfer of knowledge, skills, capacity, and power (Israel, Schulz, Parker, and Becker, 1998). Methods that are participatory in nature and allow for the transfer of knowledge and skills between the evaluators and the program beneficiaries are encouraged. Evaluators need to give explicit attention to the knowledge of community members and emphasize sharing information, decision-making power, resources, and support among members of the intervention partnership (Israel, Schulz, Parker, and Becker, 1998). Fortunately, evaluators hoping to use a more participatory approach have a large literature spanning the social sciences that has examined approaches to research in which participants are actively involved in all aspects of the research process. Examples from this literature include participatory research, participatory action research, action research, action science/inquiry, cooperative inquiry, feminist research, participatory evaluation, and empowerment evaluation (Israel, Schulz, Parker, and Becker, 1998). Common elements of these approaches include the integration of knowledge and action for the mutual benefit of all partners in the evaluation process and conducting evaluation activities in a way that promotes a co-learning and empowering process for the intended program participants (Israel, Schulz, Parker, and Becker, 1998). For evaluators, this may mean offering technical assistance to coalition members on evaluation and other skills. For example, in the East Side Village Health Worker Partnership, academic partners responsible for the evaluation responded to community requests to conduct workshops on grant writing, meeting facilitation, and questionnaire interviewing for community-based organizations involved in the project.

• *Active involvement of community members and service providers as partners is crucial in all components of the evaluation process.* A key component of any evaluation seeking to measure community capacity or related concepts is the involvement of community members and service providers in all phases of the evaluation process, including the development of the initial evaluation plan, the conceptualization of community capacity, development of instruments and interview guides, and analysis and interpretation of the data (Israel, Schulz, Parker, and Becker, 1998; Fetterman, 1994).

Although finding ways to involve community members in these processes may be challenging at times due, for example, to project outcomes stipulated at the time of funding or short time lines, involvement of project beneficiaries in identifying what is to be evaluated and how it will be evaluated can enhance the quality of the evaluation itself, as well as serve as a capacity-building exercise for all partners involved in the project. The North Carolina Community-Based Public Health Initiative evaluation was able to involve community partners in the development of the evaluation plans. Much of the first year of the project was devoted to developing the evaluation plans for each of these coalitions. The evaluation staff undertook twenty-two individual in-depth interviews and eight focus group interviews with members of each of the four coalitions. A semistructured interview guide was used, and respondents were asked "what they envisioned happening in the next four years as a result of the project" and "what would be the indicators to know that this change had happened." Results of the interviews were analyzed, and evaluation questions and indicators were identified from these interviews. Examples of indicators for one of the county coalition plans include number of registered and active voters, number of activities that health advisers are engaged in, number of agency employees undergoing cross-cultural competency training, and number of residents participating in community activities. Other indicator criteria were much more qualitative in nature, such as: "process is present for facilitating input from all community members in decision-making," "agencies give priority to problems identified by community," and "presence of organized minority health programs in health agencies."

Involving community members in the development of items for survey instruments is another important way to involve them in the evaluation process. In the East Side Village Health Worker Partnership, the steering committee was involved not only in identifying the stressors and conditioning variables used to create many of the items in the survey questionnaire, but also in decisions about the criteria to determine respondents; the recruitment, hiring, and payment of interviewers; and review of the survey instrument to suggest items to be added and deleted. (See Schulz and others, 1998, for a more detailed description of the process of developing and conducting the evaluation survey.)

One strategy for addressing the challenges of participation of all partners in the evaluation process is the joint development of some type of memorandum of understanding (Israel, Schulz, Parker, and Becker, 1998). For example, in both the East Side Village Health Worker Partnership and the Broome Team evaluations, a set of community-based public health research principles was adopted by all partners (Parker, Schulz, Israel, and Hollis, 1998; Schulz and others, 1998). The principles in use by the East Side Village Health Worker Partnership were adapted from ones earlier developed by the Detroit–Genesee County Community-Based Public Health Consortium (Schulz, Israel, Selig, and Bayer, 1998). They serve as guidelines to ensure that all research activities benefit the community and actively involve representatives of community-based organizations, public health agencies, health care organizations, and educational institutions in all major phases of the research process.

- *The use of both qualitative and quantitative methods is important.* Given the aims and the dynamic context within which community-based evaluation is conducted, methodological flexibility is essential; that is, the methods must be tailored to the purpose of the research and the context and interests of the community (Israel, Schulz, Parker, and Becker, 1998). One way to achieve this flexibility is through the use of both qualitative and quantitative methods. All four of the case examples described employ both types of data collection in their evaluation activities. Thus, these evaluations have been better able to capture the context and process, as well as the outcomes, of the interventions they are evaluating. For example, the PINAH project originally did not intend to collect qualitative data as part of the evaluation activities. But in Year 3 of the project, evaluators identified the need to incorporate qualitative interviews with residents, elected officials, community health advisers, providers, and project staff in order to amplify these respondents' perceptions and reactions about changes observed over the first four years of the project and to explain the level and direction of changes in community competence associated with the quantitative measures of health behaviors (such as service utilization) and agency collaboration (such as the pattern of referrals with community-based organizations) (Eng and Parker, 1994).

- *A strong community-based evaluator will monitor participation in the evaluation process.* Evaluations of capacity-building efforts can also contribute to monitoring, self-reflection, and modifications when necessary in the processes through which coalition members are working together. For example, a key component of the Broome Team evaluation was the development and use of the Broome Team Process Questionnaire. This instrument (adapted from an instrument developed by Israel, Schurman, Hugentobler, and House, 1992) was used to monitor collaboration among the members of the Broome Team coalition. Questions on the survey instrument asked respondents to assess their perceptions of ownership in the project, their own participation and that of others, the extent to which they felt they had influence in discussions and decision-making processes, the ability of the team to make effective decisions, and the extent to which team members felt that the Broome Team was effective in working toward change in their communities (Schulz, 1995).

Through the use of this instrument, the evaluator was able to assess how well the participatory principles of the project and the evaluation were being followed. Results from this survey were brought back to the Broome Team each year, and meeting time was set aside to discuss the results. Specific results from these assessments (reported in more detail in Schulz, 1995) were generally favorable in terms of team members' perceptions of trust and efficacy in working together. However, results were perhaps most useful as a process evaluation instrument that provided a catalyst for discussion among Broome Team members when presented as trend data, comparing results over time.

- *Timely and appropriate feedback of data to all partners throughout the project is necessary for a community-based evaluation to be successful.* Israel, Schulz, Parker, and Becker (1998) note that "community-based research seeks to disseminate findings and knowledge gained to all partners involved, in language that is understandable and respectful" (p. 180). Evaluations of community-based public health programs seeking to enhance community capacity need to do the same. Feedback of the evaluation data allows the evaluator to fulfill the requirement to be participatory in the evaluation approach. It also allows community members and service providers to discuss and interpret the evaluation data, a process that not only increases the capacity of all partners in the project but also enriches the understanding of the implications of the data results.

In the Broome Team evaluation, data from the evaluation were fed back to the team annually. Team members became engaged in the evaluation process and actively participated in discussion and interpretation of the data. As trend data became available (in Years 3 and 4 of the project), Broome Team members observed and discussed patterns in the data and used these to reflect on their own group process. For example, one year showed a drop in the generally high levels of trust reported among team members. In discussing this trend, the members identified a conflict that had emerged among members of the team in a different context, which then contributed to decreased trust within the team. Participants were able to discuss and problem-solve around this issue, and move forward in their working relationships as a result.

Future Directions

New conceptualizations of community capacity (Goodman and others, 1998; Parker and Eng, 1995) provide additional guidance for operationalizing community capacity for program and evaluation purposes. Yet much empirical work still needs to be done before evaluators know if it is possible to have one conceptual definition of community capacity and, if so, what that definition should be. However, even with these suggested new frameworks and possible future agreement on the definition of community capacity, there will always be a need to follow the participatory guidelines suggested here and to solicit community members' input in creating a vision of community capacity that is appropriate to the context of their community.

It is also important to note that the case examples here, unlike most funded health programs, were not focused on categorical diseases but rather on health broadly defined (or, in the example of the East Side Village Health Worker Partnership, the health of women and children). In addition, each of these interventions had increasing community capacity as one of its initial objectives. Projects funded to target categorical health problems may also benefit from the inclusion of intervention objectives and measures to evaluate community capacity as well as the use of more participatory methods to enhance community capacity of all project partners.

Currently, three of us are beginning interventions targeting categorical diseases. Two of us are involved with the intervention and evaluation of a household and neighborhood project seeking to reduce asthma triggers in children.

A third is involved with the development and evaluation of a lay health adviser intervention that seeks to reduce sexually transmitted diseases in a rural county. Both projects plan to include qualitative and quantitative measures of community capacity as part of their evaluation activities. The experiences of these two projects, in comparison to the four case examples described in this chapter, will provide much-needed information on the challenges and successes associated with evaluating community capacity in relationship to a categorical focused health program.

References

Brownson, R. C., Riley, P., and Bruce, T. "Demonstration Projects in Community-Based Prevention." *Journal of Public Health Management and Practice,* 1998, 4 (2), 66–77.

Cottrell, L. S. "The Competent Community." In B. H. Kaplan, R. N. Wilson, and A. H. Leighton (eds.), *Further Explorations in Social Psychiatry.* New York: Basic Books, 1976.

Eng, E., and Parker, E. "Measuring Community Competence in the Mississippi Delta: Interface Between Program Evaluation and Empowerment." *Health Education Quarterly* 1994, 21 (2), 199–220.

Eng, E., Salmon, M., and Mullan, F. "Community Empowerment: The Critical Base for Primary Health Care." *Family and Community Health,* 1992, 15 (1), 1–2.

Eng, E., and others. "Community Coalition Structures for Capacity Building: Results from the NC Community-Based Public Health Initiative." Unpublished manuscript.

Fetterman, D. M. "Empowerment Evaluation." *Evaluation Practice,* 1994, 15 (1), 1–15.

Goodman, R. M., and others. "Identifying and Defining Dimensions of Community Capacity to Provide a Basis for Measurement." *Health Education and Behavior,* 1998, 25 (3), 258–278.

Goeppinger, J., and Baglioni, A.J. "Community Competence: A Positive Approach to Needs Assessment." *American Journal of Community Psychology,* 1985, 13 (5), 507–523.

Heller, K. "The Return to Community." *American Journal of Community Psychology,* 1989, 17, 1–15.

House, J. S. *Work Stress and Social Support.* Reading, Mass.: Addison-Wesley, 1981.

Institute of Medicine. *The Future of Public Health.* Washington, D.C.: National Academy Press, 1988.

Israel, B. A., Checkoway, B., Schulz, A .J., and Zimmerman, M. A. "Health Education and Community Empowerment: Conceptualizing and Measuring Perceptions of Individual, Organizational, and Community Control." *Health Education Quarterly,* 1994, 20 (2), 149–170.

Israel, B. A., Schulz, A. J., Parker, E. A., and Becker, A. B. "Community-Based Research: A Partnership Approach to Improve Public Health." *Annual Review of Public Health,* 1998, 19, 173–202.

Israel, B. A., Cummings, M. Dignan, M. B., Heaney, C. A., Perales, D. P., Simons-Morton, B. G., and Zimmerman, M. A. "Evaluation of Health Education Programs: Current Assessment and Future Directions." *Health Education Quarterly,* 1995, 22, 364–389.

Israel, B. A., Schurman, S. J., Hugentobler, M. K., and House, J. S. "A Participatory Action Research Approach to Reducing Occupational Stress in the United States." In V. DiMartion (ed.), *Preventing Stress at Work: Conditions of Work Digest* (Vol. 2). Geneva: International Labour Office, 1992.

Katz, D., and Kahn, R. *The Social Psychology of Organizations.* New York: Wiley, 1978.

W. K. Kellogg Foundation, "Grantmaking Initiative Announcement for Community-Based Public Health." In-house document, 1990.

LaBonte, R. "Community Empowerment: The Need for Political Analysis." *Canadian Journal of Public Health,* 1989, 80, 87–88.

McKnight, J. Unpublished comments Made at Leadership and Model Development Meeting for Community-Based Public Health Initiative. Chicago: W. K. Kellogg Foundation, 1991.

McMillan, D., and Chavis, D. "Sense of Community: A Definition and Theory." *Journal of Community Psychology,* 1986, *14,* 6–23.

Parker, E. A., and Eng, E. "Conceptualizing Community Problem-Solving Capacity: Results of a Grounded Theory Study." Unpublished paper, University of Michigan, 1995.

Parker, E. A., Schulz, A. J., Israel, B. A., and Hollis, R. "East Side Detroit Village Health Worker Partnership: Community-Based Lay Health Adviser Intervention in an Urban Area." *Health Education and Behavior,* 1998, *25* (1), 24–45.

Parker, E. A., and others. "Coalition Building for Prevention: Lessons Learned from the North Carolina Community-Based Public Health Initiative." *Journal of Public Health Management and Practice,* 1998, *4* (2), 25–36.

Sampson, R. J., Raundenbush, S. W., and Earls, F. "Neighborhoods and Violent Crime: A Multilevel Study of Collective Efficacy." *Science,* 1997, *277,* 1997, 918–974.

Schulz, A. J. *Broome Team Evaluation Report.* Detroit Genesee County Community Based Public Health Project, Aug. 1994–Aug. 1995.

Schulz, A. J., Israel, B. A., Selig, S. M., and Bayer, I. S. "Development and Implementation of Principles for Community-Based Research in Public Health." In R. H. MacNair (ed.), *Research Strategies for Community Practice.* New York: Haworth Press, 1998.

Schulz, A. J., and others. "Conducting a Participatory Community-Based Survey: Collecting and Interpreting Data for a Community Health Intervention on Detroit's East Side." *Journal of Public Health Management and Practice,* 1998, *4* (2), 10–24.

Steckler, A., Dawson, L., Israel, B., and Eng, E. "Community Health Development: An Overview of the Works of Guy W. Steuart." *Health Education Quarterly,* 1993, Supplement 1, s3–s20.

Steuart, G. W. "Social and Behavioral Change Strategies." *Health Education Quarterly,* 1993, Supplement 1, s113–135.

Trostle, J. "Anthropology and Epidemiology in the 20th Century: A Selective History of Collaborative Projects and Theoretical Affinities, 1920–1970." In C. Janes and others (eds.), *Anthropology and Epidemiology.* Boston: Reidel Publishing Co., 1986.

Wallerstein, N. "Powerlessness, Empowerment, and Health: Implications for Health Promotion Programs." *American Journal of Health Promotion,* 1992, *6* (3), 197–205.

Warren, R. B., and Warren, D. I. *The Neighborhood Organizer's Handbook.* Notre Dame, Ind.: University of Notre Dame Press, 1977.

EDITH A. PARKER *is assistant professor of health behavior and health education at the University of Michigan School of Public Health.*

EUGENIA ENG *is associate professor and director of the master of public health degree program in the Department of Health Behavior and Health Education in the School of Public Health at the University of North Carolina at Chapel Hill.*

AMY J. SCHULZ *is assistant research scientist in the Department of Health Behavior and Health Education, and associate director for qualitative research for the Center on Ethnicity, Culture and Health at the University of Michigan School of Public Health.*

BARBARA A. ISRAEL *is professor and chair in the Department of Health Behavior and Health Education at the School of Public Health, University of Michigan.*

The success of a community-based program evaluation can be enhanced by using a screening tool to delineate the program's evaluative needs, resources, and commitments.

Improving the Prospects for a Successful Relationship Between Community and Evaluator

Joseph Telfair

Growth in community-based programming and the demand for valid and meaningful evaluations have fueled the need to ensure that these evaluations are conducted in a timely manner and are useful to program administrators, staff, and other community entities (Brunner and Guzman, 1989; Fawcett and others, 1996). Community projects and settings pose difficult and unique challenges in designing and implementing sound evaluations. Community-based programs usually evolve in response to a mutually recognized need by community stakeholders, with emphasis on the social, emotional, and political aspects of service delivery (Cottrell, 1976; Rothman and Tropman, 1987). Such differences in programmatic emphasis and direction may create a lack of conceptual and practical fit between service providers and evaluators. This disparity is illustrated by what one hospital-based outreach program staff person described as the difficult process of "evaluator shopping" to find an evaluator who is competent and adheres to a philosophy and orientation of service delivery methods compatible with that practiced by an organization or program (their "program theory") (Chen, 1994; Weiss, 1997).

Contours of Community-Based Evaluation

In community-based evaluation, the evaluator who serves the community has a responsibility to facilitate, support, and engage in the problem-solving aspects of these activities rather than accept definitions of activities, objectives,

I thank Jeanne Merchant and Laura Leviton for their editorial comments.

NEW DIRECTIONS FOR EVALUATION, no. 83, Fall 1999 © Jossey-Bass Publishers

or criteria that were developed by outside funders and other stakeholders. In this regard, the evaluator becomes a collaborator in the enabling process of capacity building and empowerment, ideally leading to skill development and self-determination (Fetterman, 1996; Stringer, 1996; Wallerstein, 1992). As a collaborator, the community-based program evaluator can benefit significantly from the recent expansion of work in collaborative and participatory forms of evaluation (Bailey, 1992; Cousins and Earl, 1992, 1995; Fetterman, 1996; Horsch, 1997).

Evaluation practice in community settings requires a diverse, eclectic tool-box of knowledge and skills that will allow evaluators to engage community stakeholders in a flexible yet rigorous evaluation process. The difference between community-based evaluation and other types of evaluation lies in understanding and accommodating the situation or fit of communities, of their leadership, and their perception of needs—termed the *cultural reality* of communities. This distinction has its intellectual foundation in ecological psychology.

Evaluators become involved with community-based programs by being asked to be the outside evaluator by an authoritative person at the federal, state, or local level; by asking to become involved (for example, in response to a grant announcement); or as part of the community team, adding the target problem to their evaluation agenda (Herman, Morris, and Fitz-Gibbon, 1987; Rossi and Freeman, 1993; Whyte, Greenwood, and Lazes, 1991). How evaluators become involved usually dictates the evaluative approach (formative or summative), design (experimental, quasi-experimental, or something else), and model (traditional or community-based) they will use. Evaluators may recognize that a more participatory and collaborative evaluation is needed in the community-based setting, but there is concern that the scientific rigor of evaluations produced with such models might be compromised (Cousins and others, 1996; Weiss, 1983). Community programs need engagement with an evaluation approach that is eclectic, flexible (allowing for as needed changes), integrative of relevant concepts and components from existing evaluation models, incorporative of scientifically sound principles, and balanced, maintaining the integrity and rigor that evaluators have demanded for the past three decades. From work with a number of small to moderate-sized service-oriented programs, we have learned that lack of evaluation engagement may result in unplanned and unavoidable difficulties as the evaluation process progresses.

Successful Community-Based Evaluations

One of the primary concerns that evaluators of community programs and agencies have is to ensure that the evaluation endeavor is deemed mutually successful by the evaluators themselves and by the community entity. It is understood that to achieve this assurance, engagement in a process of negotiation toward clarity of purpose for the evaluation, as well as its expected results, tasks, and outcomes, is required. For our purposes this process is termed *front loading the evaluation*. It is part of the planning and preevaluation assessment and is based on the concepts that underlie the performance of an evaluability assessment (Rossi and Freeman, 1993; Wholey, 1987). Although used primarily at the state and national levels, this technique can be adapted for use at the local level (Leviton, Collins, Laird, and Kratt, 1998). Evaluability assessment is a set of procedures that includes and takes into account the interest of community entities in order to maximize the utility of the evaluation (Rossi and Freeman, 1993). This type of assessment necessitates a participatory or collaborative approach to arrive at the ultimate goal of clarifying the intended use of the evaluation information. For our purposes, this assessment is likely to contribute to the following:

A helpful solving of problems that might otherwise inhibit useful community-based evaluation
Directions for improved program performance or success
A clarification of the program's intent from the point of view of the community entity
An exploration of the cultural reality of the program to clarify the plausibility of stated objectives and the "feasibility of performance measurement" or achievement of these objectives (Wholey, 1987)
An assessment of the likelihood of a good fit between the evaluators' talents and the communities' perceived needs for, commitment to, and use of evaluation (Patton, 1997).

In regard to the last, in our experience with several rural social and health services programs serving African Americans, we have found that additional labor must be put into understanding and achieving this fit if the evaluation effort is to have a chance of succeeding. However, given the unique and varied nature, function, and characteristics of community entities and the circumstances under which evaluators are engaged with them, this front loading does not always occur in a timely manner. The consequence of this delay is a diminution of the relationship between community entity and evaluator and the potential success of the evaluation process.

We have observed that the demand for accountability of community-based services and related programs has been spurred by the growing emphasis of public and private funders (mostly foundations) on outcome-based community service programs. As one executive director of a twenty-five-year-old community-based program serving African Americans stated, "They [foundations] know we have done it and can do it [effectively serve clients], but now they want us to prove it. So we need help." We have also observed an exponential increase in requests for assistance in community-based evaluations. As a result, we developed the Evaluation Pre-Screening Tool (EPST), which is used prior to finalizing evaluation agreements and allows for the assessment of the likelihood of a good fit between the evaluators' talents and the communities' perceived commitment to, and needs and resources for, evaluation. In short, it allows both to come to a mutual agreement as to the feasibility of conducting an evaluation of a program or service and to lay the groundwork designed to increase the probable success of such an endeavor.

Review of the many returned EPSTs has taught us that the logical order of the questions should move from a descriptive overview of the existing program and its services to a description of the anticipated evaluation assistance that will be needed. In addition, the order of the questions is designed to help the community entity focus, going from the broad generalizations of the program or service area to specifics about what is needed. The latter is something that should occur but often does not when evaluators work with community-based programs.

Use of the Evaluation Pre-Screening Tool

Community entities are asked to complete the EPST in reference to those who are, or are expected to be, involved with the project(s) (when possible). Throughout the EPST document, the involved staff are referred to as "YOUR TEAM." We make this request because most often when the evaluator is asked to provide assistance to community-based programs, it is the program or executive director who provides him or her with the information to plan and implement the evaluation. The problem is that these staff members are not responsible for the agency's or program's "grunt" work (for example, provision of services to clients, recruitment of clients, interviewing clients using evaluation data forms). Also, if the project is a collaborative one, these executive or program directors may lack adequate information on the functions, resources, and politics of their collaborators. The line (nonadministrative) staffs do the "grunt work." Our experience suggests that because of the size, nature, structure, and function of many of these community-based programs, the line staffs are very aware of and involved in the day-to-day issues of the program or agency. Leaving them out of the initial planning constrains their buy-in to the eventual plan and may result in the exclusion of key insights, causing difficulties at different points in the evaluation process. In addition, we have found that because change is the one constant for community entities, initial agreements of understanding between potential collaborators often have to be adjusted as the particulars of projects are finalized. Excluding these collaborators (or their representatives) can also lead to potential implementation difficulties down the line.

The EPST's three sections describe the existing programs and services, the programs and services to be included in the proposed evaluation collaboration, and the proposed program and services that will be needed to develop and maintain the proposed evaluation collaboration. In addition, we include a list of logistical and related information that will be needed. We list potential agreements that may or will be needed to bring closure to the decision phase of the preassessment process, which may not have been covered, in the main body of the EPST. After each question, blank lines are provided for the recording of responses arrived at by the team. The respondents are told to use extra pages if needed. Also, respondents are asked to provide additional materials (for example, brochures, reports) that would help clarify the nature, scope, content area, and history of the program and the services it provides.

Because not all programs are of the same type, have the same focus or purpose, or have the same reasons for asking for evaluation assistance, the questions within the EPST are slightly modified for fit. For example, one program to which we were asked to provide assistance resided within a large state-level institution that had many layers of bureaucracy, from which approval was needed in order for work to get done. In the second section of the EPST, we usually ask the potential collaborators to describe the resources they would have available to support the evaluation effort. In most cases this question is answered in relation to personnel, financial (most often outside funders), and community supports; however, in the case of this program, we had to be more specific and add a question about the internal administrative support for the program's evaluation plans. In such institutions, a vision at the program level may not be shared at the institutional level. It is at the institutional level where the final approval for the program's going forward with any innovations or changes must be approved. Therefore, any evaluation efforts, no matter how carefully conceived or rigorously planned, can be disapproved for many reasons, some of which have nothing to do with the program. Unfortunately this is what happened in the case of the program mentioned above. One of the reasons for disapproval was that those at the higher administrative level did not want to invest any additional funds in it. By discovering this early on, all involved were clear that the consultation had to be delayed until the issue of financial support from the institution was resolved.

After the completed EPST is returned and analyzed, the evaluator provides verbal and written feedback to the community entity for the purpose of providing an appraisal of the status of the program and its services, clarifying the goal and objectives of the program for all involved, and providing information that will allow agencies or programs to decide if they want to discontinue the evaluation consultation, delay the consultation, or proceed with the consultation and, if so, at what level (for example, conduct a needs and asset assessment only or conduct a summative or a formative evaluation). Entities generally complete the EPST within 1 to 2 meetings. The results are then mailed to the evaluator, who reviews them in preparation for further work.

EPST Section I: Description of Existing Programs and Services. In this section, community entities are asked to provide the evaluator with a descriptive overview of its existing programs and services. This information assists the evaluator in gaining a critical understanding of the existing structural, social, political, and historical approach to, or philosophy of, service aspects and components of the target program or service. We ask community entities to address the following six questions, reminding them that for each question they are to answer in reference to those who are, or are expected to be, involved with the project ("YOUR TEAM"):

1. What are the critical/core activities, staffing, and administrative arrangements, etc. of your current program(s)?
2. How many participants (average # of clients) and staff (by type/title) are taking part in the programs/agencies activities? (*Please include in your answer* a summary of staff roles and specific activities clients take the lead or play a major role in—for example, consumer advisory councils.)
3. Which parts of the current program does your team consider its most distinctive characteristics (for example, its staff, location, type of clientele, etc.)—those that make it unique among programs of its kind? (*Please include in your answer* the distinctive characteristics of all those who would be participating in the proposed project.)
4. Who are your typical contact persons or agencies (collaborators) and what is your administrative relationship with them? That is, is there direct or indirect accountability with your office? Is your program a decentralized (autonomous of the health department or other funding agency) or centralized (direct responsibility to the health department or other funding agency) one?
5. Given that your program provides multiple types of services, how do the program components vary (if at all) (describe each: purpose, tasks and expected outcomes)? (*In your reply please include* the primary person(s) responsible for each component and the length of time this(ese) person(s) had worked with this(ese) components.)
6. (a) What are the goals of your current program? (b) What objectives and subobjectives are essential to the attainment of program goals? and (c) What gaps exist in the attainment of objectives or subobjectives?

A case example illustrates the need for these questions. In one project aimed at providing health outreach services to citizens in a small rural county, we did not use the questions contained in this section of the EPST in our planning with the lead agency. This agency had commitments from a number of past collaborating agencies to work with it on this recently funded federal project. These collaborators were not just co-service agencies, but because of the size of the county, members of the administrative staff work on committees and task forces, and many socialized with each other on a regular basis. A key component of the project's first year was to conduct a summative evaluation that would include the gathering of data to establish base rates for a list of health conditions and health and social services. These data were to be used to determine clients' health conditions and access to, and use of, health and social services that were to be the targets of the funded intervention.

The plan was to conduct surveys on a random-probability sample of households to gather this information. All of the preparation for this task was carried out between the evaluator and the lead agency, as was agreed on by the project's collaborators. It was an innovation of the grant that a local evaluation committee consisting of representatives from each of the collaborators and some consumers developed the data collection survey tool. However, members of the local team reported to, but were not members of, the executive committee who oversaw and made decisions about the functioning of the project. It was never clear how much the executive committee understood about the first phase of the project, which would have been a key area of discussion if the first section of EPST questions had been used. Thus, when it came to implementation of the survey, none of the collaborators, save one, was involved. The primary reason for this lack of involvement was the fact that executive committee members had not thought through the resources they would need to commit to this phase of the project. They had given their verbal and conceptual support to the project, but found they could not meet their required in-kind contributions.

As a consequence, the lead agency and the evaluator had to draw up an alternative plan for a reduced sample size. The administrative staffs of the collaborators were only peripherally rather than fully engaged in the dialogue regarding the logistics of carrying out the well-laid-out assessment plan developed by the local evaluation committee. Therefore, the details of what they would need to contribute were significantly underestimated. Despite the close working relationship that collaborators had with one another, because they did not fully explore or get questioned about the existing resources and capacities, implementation problems occurred at a point in the early stages of the project.

Of course, there is no guarantee that all resource problems would have been avoided by asking the questions in section I of the EPST, but the exploration process might have proved worthwhile in anticipating them and thus planning in advance how to address them.

EPST Section II: Description of Program and Services. In this section, community entities are asked to provide the evaluator with a description of the rationale, goals, and objectives of the program; the potential evaluation; and the focused program or service areas of the potential evaluation. Information on the resources available to support the evaluation is also requested. This information assists the entity and the evaluator in gaining a critical understanding of the level of forethought and planning prior to seeking the consultation.

This set of questions provides a road map for the work that is to be carried out and the extent to which the work can be accomplished. Potential collaborators are asked to examine and discuss both internal and external supports and barriers. Issues of maintenance and sustainability of effort are addressed. In this section of the EPST we ask community entities to address the following five questions:

1. *In relation to the proposed program evaluation collaboration:* (a) What component(s) of the program would your team like the proposed evaluation collaboration to address? (b) What will the proposed evaluation collaboration add? Do you see these as short- or long-term additions? (c) How will the components of the proposed evaluation/research collaboration be integrated into your existing program?

2. *In relation to the proposed evaluation collaboration:* Why does your team think evaluation collaboration is needed? That is, what is your team's rationale for what makes it important, who will benefit, and why?

3. *In relation to the proposed evaluation collaboration:* (a) What does your team see as the primary goals of the evaluation collaboration? (b) What objectives and subobjectives does your team think are essential to the attainment of the evaluation collaboration goals? and (c) What are the anticipated short- and long-range outcomes (or impact) of the proposed evaluation/research collaboration? That is, what does your team hope the institution of the proposed evaluation consultation will accomplish?

4. *In relation to the evaluation collaboration:* (a) What does your team anticipate as the supports (for example, resources or politics, etc.) for the development and maintenance of the proposed evaluation collaboration beyond the initial term? (b) What are the anticipated obstacles (for example, political, technical, or logistical, etc.) to the evaluation collaboration's development and maintenance (long-term evaluation collaboration)?

5. *In relation to the proposed evaluation collaboration:* (a) What does your team see as the central activities related to the proposed evaluation collaboration? (b) What resources (for example, budget, personnel) and materials (for example, on-site computers, other equipment) does your team anticipate to be available to carry out the evaluation collaboration activities?

EPST Section III: Description of Program and Services. In this section, community entities are asked to provide the evaluator with a description of the assistance they anticipate will be needed from the evaluator. Entities are asked to be as thorough as possible, basing their answer on their team's understanding of what will be needed to develop and maintain the proposed evaluation collaboration. Although this section assists the evaluator by asking the entity to describe why it needs help from the evaluation consultant, it usually brings up important questions for the entity itself, such as the qualifications, ability, potential compatibility (fit), and requested resources by the evaluator (for example, personnel and financing). We have found that often the evaluator is requested in order to get some clarity on what can and cannot be asked for. This is particularly true for small to moderate-sized programs that have limited funds to spend on the evaluation.

At the community-based program level, many are beginning to understand the need for data from sound evaluations that can justify or support the existence of their program or the services it delivers. We have found, however, that these community entities do not understand what resources (personnel or financial) are needed in order to conduct even a basic evaluation. Many have had to scale back the level of their request because they lack the resources.

For example, a community-based service agency serving persons with a hematalogic blood disorder was asked by one of its hospital-based charity funders to conduct an efficacy study of one of its home health services. This was a first for the agency, and our evaluation team was asked to assist since we have had a five-year relationship with it. Meetings were conducted to clarify goals and objectives, what service components were to be assessed, why the funder was interested in these particular services, what was known about the services (from the literature, previous assessments, and the agency's experience to date), what the expected outcomes of the assessment were, and what resources were available to conduct such an endeavor. The community-based agency made it very clear that it did not want the assessment to be a "research study that gives us nothing we can use." The funders' expectations, however, translated into the need for a randomized control trial that would involve resources the agency did not have and was not initially willing to provide, as well as a sample size that was much larger than any obtainable by the agency.

To reconcile this difference, the evaluator used information gathered from the first two sections of the EPST, as well as being aided by a history with the agency and the background information on home health services provided at the community level, and with conducting rigorous assessments at the community level. At a follow-up meeting, a compromise was reached: the funders agreed to a quasi-experimental design (using quantitative and qualitative methods) that integrated their concerns with the agency's need for applied information. The agency's administrator was also able to get the funder to provide moderate support for the new design, reassign staff to assist with the special project, and allow staff to work with the evaluator to determine the most appropriate indicators and targets that would be needed for as rigorous an assessment as possible.

EPST Section IV: Needed Logistical and Related Information. Based on early pilot testing, we found that more facts are often needed to bring closure to the front-loading process, which may not be contained in the documentation from the previous three sections of the EPST. Therefore, the closing section of the EPST contains a list of logistical and related information that is needed to allow for agreements and decisions to be made that concludes the decision phase of the consultation. This list may be modified to address the unique characteristics of the program under consideration. The most common elements of the list that are requested (or to be considered) are as follows:

1. A description of the questions that will be addressed based on the collected data.
2. A description of the primary goals and objectives of the program.
3. The data collection methods you have planned, including sources, site, instruments or other data collection methods.
4. A time line for all planning, development, and maintenance of assessment and evaluation consultation activities.
5. An understanding and list of the tasks and responsibilities that program staff or others involved will undertake.
6. A schedule of required reports to and meetings with stakeholders (including auxiliary staffs, clients, and the community).
7. The budget available for planning, development, and long-term maintenance, and other anticipated costs of the program, as well as the evaluation consultation.

8. In line with the expected outcomes, a plan describing the best use of the collected data in the service of the clients and for other programmatic purposes (for example, grant development).
9. An outline of the services and assistance the evaluation team can provide.

Conclusion

In the use of the EPST, our focus is primarily on small to moderate-sized service-oriented programs and agencies; however, we have used it with programs and agencies of all sizes and types. Although no approach is perfect, the use of the EPST has resulted in about an 85 percent rate of achieving the evaluation process outcomes described above. Results from use of the EPST commonly fall into four broad categories:

- For a number of reasons (for example, limited funding, uneven commitment of personnel or administration, lack of political will) the community entity is not ready to engage in evaluation at the present time or at all.
- The EPST helped the community entity clarify, redefine, or confirm the goals and objectives of the program, and, as one director of an urban, hospital-based, teenage pregnancy-prevention program stated, "It helped us confirm why we started this program in the first place."
- Planned evaluation will need to be placed on hold until issues or problems influencing the community entity's ability to engage in the evaluation process are resolved.
- What the community entity really wanted was either something less than an evaluation (for example, program monitoring or a needs assessment) or a specific type of evaluation (for example, a summative assessment of specific data or a longitudinal assessment that is parallel with the planned growth and development of the targeted program or one of its services).

Our experience suggests that many of the community-based entities find the EPST results helpful, since often these programs do not have the time or resources to conduct or obtain a professional audit.

References

Bailey, D. "Using Participatory Research in Community Consortia Development and Evaluation: Lessons from the Beginning of a Story." *American Sociologist,* 1992, *23,* 71–82.

Brunner, I., and Guzman, A. "Participatory Evaluation: A Tool to Assess and Empower People." In R. F. Connor and M. H. Hendricks (eds.), *International Innovations in Evaluation Methodology.* New Directions for Program Evaluation, no. 42. San Francisco: Jossey-Bass, 1989.

Chen, H. T. "Theory-Driven Evaluations: Needs, Difficulties, and Options." *Evaluation Practice,* 1994, *15,* 79–82.

Cottrell Jr., L. S. "The Competent Community." In B. H. Kaplan, R. N. Wilson, and A. H. Leighton (eds.), *Further Explorations in Social Psychiatry.* New York: Basic Books, 1976.

Cousins, J. B. "Consequences of Researcher Involvement in Participatory Evaluation." *Studies in Educational Evaluation,* 1996, *22* (1), 3–27.

Cousins, J. B., and Earl, L. M. "The Case for Participatory Evaluation." *Educational Evaluation and Policy Analysis,* 1992, *14,* 533–538.

Cousins, J. B., and Earl, L. M. "The Case for Participatory Evaluation: Theory, Research, Practice." In J. B. Cousins and L. M. Earl (eds.), *Participatory Evaluation in Education: Studies in Evaluation Use and Organizational Learning.* London: Palmer Press, 1995.

Cousins, J. B., Donahue, J. J., and Bloom, G. A. "Collaborative Evaluation in North America: Evaluators' Self-Reported Opinions, Practices, and Consequences." *Evaluation Practice,* 1996, *17,* 207–226.

Fawcett, S., and others. "Empowering Community Health Initiatives Through Evaluation." In D. Fetterman, S. Kaftarian, and A. Wandersman (eds.), *Empowerment Evaluation: Knowledge and Tools for Self-Assessment and Accountability.* Thousand Oaks, Calif.: Sage, 1996.

Fetterman, D. "Empowerment Evaluation: An Introduction to Theory and Practice." In D. Fetterman, S. J. Kaftarian, and A. Wandersman (eds.), *Empowerment Evaluation: Knowledge and Tools for Self-Assessment and Accountability.* Thousand Oaks, Calif.: Sage, 1996.

Herman, J. L., Morris, L. L., and Fitz-Gibbon, C. T. *Evaluator's Handbook.* Thousand Oaks, Calif.: Sage, 1987.

Horsch, K. (1997). "Evaluating CBIs: Facing the Challenge and Improving Practice." *Evaluation Exchange,* 1997, *3* (3/4), 1–7.

Leviton, L. C., Collins, C. B., Laird, B. L., and Kratt, P. P. "Teaching Evaluation Using Evaluability Assessment." *Evaluation,* 1998, *4* (4), 389–409.

Patton, M. Q. *Utilization-Focused Evaluation.* (3rd ed.) Thousand Oaks, Calif.: Sage, 1997.

Rossi, P. H., and Freeman, H. E. *Evaluation: A Systematic Approach* (5th ed.) Thousand Oaks, Calif.: Sage, 1993.

Rothman, J., and Tropman, J. E. "Models of Community Organization and Macro Practice Perspectives: Their Mixing and Phasing." In F. M. Cox, J. L. Erlich, J. Rothman, and J. E. Tropman (eds.), *Strategies of Community Organization: Macro Practice.* Itasca, Ill.: Peacock, 1987.

Stringer, E. T. *Action Research: A Handbook for Practitioners.* Thousand Oaks, Calif.: Sage, 1996.

Wallerstein, N. "Powerlessness, Empowerment and Health: Implications for Health Promotion Programs." *American Journal of Health Promotion,* 1992, *6,* 197–204.

Weiss, C. H. "The Stakeholder Approach to Evaluation: Origins and Promise." In A. S. Byrk (ed.), *Stakeholder-Based Education.* New Directions for Program Evaluation, no. 17. San Francisco: Jossey-Bass, 1983.

Weiss, C. H. "Theory-Based Evaluation: Past, Present and Future." In Rog, D. J., and Fournier, D. (eds.), *Progress and Future Directions in Evaluation: Perspectives on Theory, Practice, and Methods.* New Directions for Evaluation, no. 76. San Francisco: Jossey-Bass, 1997.

Wholey, J. S. "Evaluability Assessment: Developing Program Theory." In L. Bickman (ed.), *Using Program Theory in Evaluation.* New Directions for Program Evaluation, no. 33. San Francisco: Jossey-Bass, 1987.

Whyte, W. F., Greenwood, D. J., and Lazes, P. "Participatory Action Research: Through Practice to Science in Social Research." In W. F. Whyte (ed.), *Participatory Action Research.* Thousand Oaks, Calif.: Sage, 1991.

JOSEPH TELFAIR is associate professor in the Department of Maternal and Child Health, School of Public Health and Director, Division of Social, Health Services and Community-Based Research within the Comprehensive Sickle Cell Center, School of Medicine, at the University of Alabama at Birmingham.

*The Robert Wood Johnson Foundation sponsors the Fighting
Back initiative, in which communities across the country
receive funding to combat alcohol and drug use. The evaluators
of this initiative have tried to present an evaluation that is
responsive to both national policy agendas and local
community contextual differences, and thus offer important
insight for both levels.*

The View from Main Street and the View from 40,000 Feet: Can a National Evaluation Understand Local Communities?

Leonard Saxe, Elizabeth Tighe

As evaluators, we take it as a given that programs need data to determine whether their efforts have been effective. Local communities are taking greater control and responsibility for program design and implementation. Therefore, evaluators need to achieve a better balance between efforts that develop valid conclusions that can be replicated across situations and time and conclusions that are of immediate import to sustain or maintain the program. For policy-making, our goal in evaluating local programs remains a synthesis of results to distill underlying principles about behavior and community change. These can then be applied to other communities. At the same time, involving community leaders can increase the sensitivity of the evaluation to local issues, and thus make the evaluation more useful. Our evaluation of Fighting Back exemplifies such an effort.

This chapter describes an approach to incorporating two models of evaluation: an accountability model and an empowerment model. Our focus is how both to stand back from a program and view it objectively, while also being on the ground and helping to collect data that can be used to develop and support the program implementation. The scientific accountability model of evaluation has its roots in efforts from the Great Society era to make social programs accountable. A model of evaluation based on scientific methods evolved whereby social programs were viewed as "treatments" that were compared over time or to comparison groups (Campbell, 1969; Saxe and Fine, 1981). Although there has been criticism of the model, it does address the questions of external audiences concerning the outcome of policies. This model has always existed in tension with efforts to empower those with responsibility for program development and implementation (Fetterman, 1996; Patton, 1978; Stake, 1975). The tension is increasingly evident as accountability is enforced and, at the same time, decision-making reverts to those with direct program responsibility.

Devolution of responsibility to the local level has been key to social innovation in government and social services since the 1970s. Programs that were formerly designed and managed by the federal government are now bloc-granted to states and local agencies. Local communities have a new set of responsibilities; no longer merely held accountable for managing programs, they are now responsible for how the program is designed and implemented. Thus, for example, substance abuse policy has increasingly focused on the development of community-based programs to reduce demand for drugs and to implement comprehensive identification and treatment services (Office of National Drug Control Policy, 1998; Winick and Larson, 1997). Community representatives involved in such programs need evaluative feedback to manage their initiatives. Yet community representatives are not the only stakeholders; in particular, policymakers need to know if these types of programs are effective. Serving both sets of stakeholders is a significant challenge; however, we have discovered that their needs can be compatible. For evaluation to be effective, it needs to satisfy the mutual interests of communities and national sponsors.

To illustrate the synergy between local and national perspectives, we focus here on the Fighting Back program of the Robert Wood Johnson Foundation (RWJF). Fighting Back is the first national demonstration of communitywide substance abuse prevention (Jellinek and Hearn, 1991; Spickard, Dixon, and Sarver, 1994). Communities designed site-specific approaches to reduce the demand for alcohol and other drugs (AOD) and related harms. This was accomplished by developing coalitions among public agencies, private organizations, and citizens' groups. These groups were charged with developing and implementing a comprehensive plan to deploy AOD programs across the continuum of care in their community, including public awareness, prevention, early identification, treatment, and aftercare.

Local control over program design and implementation was central to the Fighting Back initiative. The theory behind Fighting Back employed several assumptions about communities. First, each community was assumed to have unique characteristics that affected the nature of its substance abuse problem. Second, effective programming was believed to be more likely when grassroots leaders increased communication with managers of programs (including health care, social services, and police) than when external experts, unfamiliar with the local context, imposed their solutions. Citizens needed to be involved in the development of solutions in order to change communitywide attitudes and behavior about substance use and misuse. In addition, emphasis was placed on local control because external solutions had focused almost exclusively on supply reduction (reducing the availability of drugs) rather than on demand reduction (reducing the desire for drugs). At the time Fighting Back was conceived, the nation was witnessing high levels of inner-city crime associated with substance abuse—in particular, violence associated with the use and sale of crack cocaine (Jellinek and Hearn, 1991; Musto, 1992). Reducing demand was perceived as key, but no models existed to reduce both supply and demand at the community level.

Although the demonstration was designed to test a new model of prevention, the program was developed in communities that were already experimenting with ways to deal with substance abuse. Not uncommon for evaluation studies, the difference in focus between the policymakers and the community leaders created tension that evaluators often felt. Tension between the policymakers' need for causal information and local stakeholders' concern for supportive feedback underlay the evaluation of Fighting Back. These two concerns had to be balanced by the evaluation design.

Although Fighting Back is a national initiative funded by a private philanthropy, it has many government parallels. Among the substance abuse prevention programs, the Community Partnership Programs of the Center for Substance Abuse Prevention (1996) are the most prominent and probably most similar to Fighting Back. Through this initiative, over 250 partnerships were awarded up to five years of funding. Typically partnerships served entire counties, although some served smaller areas. The ultimate goal of these programs was to change the community in such a way that everyone would feel responsibility toward, and be involved in, preventing substance abuse. Other drug prevention programs supported by the national government include D.A.R.E, Drug Free Communities, and various efforts to reduce crime and other harms associated with drug use (Winick and Larson, 1997).

Validity Versus Utility

The evaluation of locally controlled programs, such as the Fighting Back demonstration, requires integrating models focused on validity with those focused on utility. Shadish, Cook, and Leviton (1991) characterize the differences between these models in terms of the experimenting society (Campbell, 1969, 1988), explanatory theorists (Cronbach, 1982; Weiss, 1977), and stakeholder models (Patton, 1978, 1997; Stake, 1975, 1980; Wholey, 1983). Each of these perspectives has strengths and weaknesses. Although evaluators recognize that greater consideration should be given to a model of evaluation that combines the three perspectives, they rarely do so. Typically evaluators adopt a single perspective, and they emphasize either validity or utility. The evaluation of Fighting Back tried to maximize both validity and utility and to play to the strengths across models rather than the differences between them. The emphasis is on truth and objectivity in evaluation rather than advocacy (Scriven, 1997).

Well-designed experiments maximizing internal validity have been important to the development of alcohol, tobacco, and other drugs (ATOD) programs. For example, in the mid-1980s, amid growing concern about the use of alcohol, drugs, and tobacco by youth, Botvin and colleagues developed the Life Skills Program designed to strengthen students' abilities to resist peer and social influences to use ATOD (Botvin, Baker, Filazzola and Botvin, 1990). In 1985 dozens of schools in New York State were randomly assigned either to receive or not receive this program. Six years later, students who had participated in the Life Skills Program showed significantly lower rates of substance use than comparison group counterparts (Botvin and others, 1995). These studies appear to have good internal validity, but some threats still exist because of the context.

The Life Skills Program cannot occur without all of those involved (students, teachers, school administrators) knowing about its desired consequences. Students reported lower rates of substance use on standard questionnaires, but the specific effects of the Life Skills Program cannot be separated from the additional effects of fifteen hour-long education sessions for teachers and other adults. As Campbell (1971) noted, the added variation introduced by the social context will inevitably be confounded with the intervention, making it difficult to interpret observed outcomes, regardless of randomization.

Given that a completely unbiased social experiment appears infeasible, alternative models, such as the explanatory and stakeholder models, seek to emphasize utility in evaluative research. These models emphasize the complexity of social problems in their context. Rather than studying simple causal relationships between a limited number of controllable variables, evaluation should model the complexity of social problems as they exist in the social world. This includes gaining better understanding of why a program might yield positive results in some contexts and no results or reverse effects in others by explaining higher-order interactions, emphasizing external validity over internal validity (Cronbach, 1982; Chen and Rossi, 1983; Weiss, 1978). It also includes evaluations that are of immediate and direct use to those involved in implementing the programs (Patton, 1978; Stake, 1975, 1980; Wholey, 1983). For example, despite possible problems with the interpretation of causality associated with the Life Skills Program, the intervention appears to provide many benefits to the students who participated (Botvin and others, 1995; Hawkins, Catalano, and Miller, 1992; Tobler, 1986; Tobler and Stratton, 1997). We may not understand why the program is effective, but the data make clear that whatever is done is useful. That is, under certain conditions, positive effects are obtained, regardless of what underlying construct might have been manipulated.

This emphasis on the utility of evaluative research regardless of the level of experimental rigor is best represented in the stakeholder models of evaluation. The pinnacle of this evaluation perspective is perhaps represented in current discussions of empowerment evaluation (Fetterman, Kaftarian, and Wandersman, 1996). Fetterman (1996) describes empowerment evaluation as having its roots in community psychology. Thus, it is understandable that this perspective has gained prominence as social programs become more locally or community based. Empowerment, however, described as facilitating self-determination through evaluation, is similar to the more utilitarian models of the 1970s (Patton, 1978; Stake, 1975, 1980; Wholey, 1983). Called responsiveness models or management-centered models, their focus has been on making evaluation useful.

Although evaluation research needs to be useful, to the extent that evaluation becomes confounded with program implementation, the greater are the threats to the validity of the evaluation process (Scriven, 1997). Evaluation does not have to be valid in order for it to be useful, or at least perceived to be useful. Thus, for example, Beveridge and others (forthcoming) have described how data from the National Household Survey on Drug Abuse were used to show that the Miami Coalition Against Drug Abuse had reduced substance use by 50 percent. The finding was touted in advertisements and prompted a visit by President Clinton to Miami to declare victory in the war against drugs. Unfortunately, the finding was artifactual. It was most likely the result of Hurricane Andrew. The hurricane devastated parts of the target area and made it impossible to sample similar households after the storm.

Fighting Back

Fighting Back has contended with the balance issue throughout its history: how to hold sites accountable to objective standards of program effectiveness, while being supportive of and sensitive to their ongoing program development. The national evaluation of this program was implemented primarily as an outcome evaluation: the ultimate question to be answered was whether rates of AOD use, and harms from use, declined significantly in the communities in which the program was implemented (Rindskopf and Saxe, 1998; Saxe and others, 1997). We employed a quasi-experimental design to examine twelve of the Fighting Back communities, along with thirty matched comparison communities. We developed standardized measures of use and harm that could be used and analyzed across all communities. These included both a random-digit-dial survey and archival indicators, such as crime data and mortality. In addition to these standardized outcome measures, the evaluation included in-depth ethnographic studies in several of the communities and a management information system implemented in all twelve Fighting Back communities to track program implementation.

Fighting Back then moved into a new phase with additional funding for eight of the communities participating in the project. At this point, assessment specific to localities and deemed useful became increasingly important in the evaluation. Communities needed local data for their own planning. Future funding became dependent on a community's ability to assess its progress in achieving reductions in AOD use and harm. Toward this end, the funder required sites to develop community reporting systems, modeled after community epidemiological working groups (CEWG). The data were intended to assess community progress in achieving AOD and harm reductions, but also for local planning.

The new phase of Fighting Back has altered the role and use of data. Not only do the sites and evaluators now have different interests, but also the evaluators and program managers have increasingly different concerns. The evaluators are concerned with drawing valid inferences about the program, while the program managers must ensure that the sites do well. Sites now seek to report local outcome levels. To address this problem, both the evaluators and program managers must be attuned to motives that can influence data collection and possibly lead to confounders. The need for the national evaluation became more directly involved in the local evaluation process. Some of the local data are a subset of the national evaluation data. Other locally specific information is not collected by the national evaluation and must be acquired and analyzed locally. Portions of these data are necessary for the national evaluation but need to be collected by the local community in collaboration with national evaluators. Thus, local assessment from the national evaluation perspective takes several forms, and each form has different implications for the evaluation and for the participating communities.

National Evaluation Data. Although collected in a common form across sites, the national data disaggregated to individual communities have potentially important utility for planning. Communities need assistance in gaining access to these data, interpreting the results, and using them appropriately to identify and respond to their communities' substance abuse problems. The interpretation and appropriate-use issues are significant, especially in the context of national-level survey samples that require different weighting schemes when examined at local levels. Policymakers have perhaps overemphasized "scorecarding" substance abuse rates; often scorecards ignore the context of a community and the extraneous factors that affect AOD use and attitudes. Also, random changes in substance use rates make them complex to use. Survey and indicator findings become inappropriate to compare. Finally, most of the national measures became available only after a considerable lag. The national data can provide rapid feedback only under limited circumstances. Nevertheless, the evaluators were in a position to help communities use the available survey and indicator data in their planning.

Locally Collected Data. The national evaluation was designed to test the concept that communitywide strategies could address the prevention and treatment of substance abuse. For this reason, we sought measures of the use and harm caused by substance abuse that could be assessed across the communities. Each community may offer unique and important data—unique, at least, in terms of how they are collected. School surveys of drug and alcohol attitudes and behavior can illustrate the issues. For both practical and legal reasons, it is infeasible for the national evaluation to collect its own data through school surveys (Hunt, 1998). Most communities, however, conduct school surveys or would be interested in doing so. The data from these surveys can provide essential information about the impact of Fighting Back. The national evaluators therefore supported communities in conducting their own surveys through technical assistance and material resources, if needed. Because the surveys are locally controlled, it is likely that each will use slightly different instruments and designs. The evaluators can use the data and deal with the differences in instruments by applying meta-analytic techniques. The school survey situation may be unique; in other cases—for example, data about school dropouts or criminal activity—locally collected data would not be used directly by the national evaluation. It would be important, though, for the national evaluation to be involved in the development of such studies to ensure quality and avoid conflicts with other data collection activities. If successful, these efforts could provide important and timely information about the impact of Fighting Back.

Evaluation of Specific Initiatives. The Fighting Back program concept does not specify which interventions particular communities will adopt. Interventions may change frequently, in both their specifics and the role of Fighting Back. It is important and useful for communities to evaluate these interventions. The national evaluation team can help to ensure that these studies are likely to yield valid and useful information.

The new role for evaluation data for this phase of Fighting Back has several implications. Most important, the need has become acute to maintain independence between the evaluation and program functions. If they are constrained by a need to "make the program look good," the evaluators cannot conduct an objective assessment and provide evidence that will convince skeptical policymakers of the value of Fighting Back. Our position therefore is that the evaluators need to be responsible for working with communities on local assessment issues. Where appropriate, the evaluators would provide data, analyses, and technical assistance.

We have also sought to infuse locally driven data collection efforts with the type of objective standards applied at the national level. We worked with communities' questions about local data to focus on the three key principles: validity, utility, and feasibility. *Validity* means these data should measure what the underlying constructs intend. *Utility* means the data must also be useful to one or more of the stakeholder groups. Although they cannot always determine this a priori, both evaluators and community members should think through how they might use the findings. Finally, the data must be feasible to collect. *Feasibility* encompasses two considerations: whether the measure is likely to be sensitive to detecting change reliably (that is, effect sizes are likely to show statistically significant change) and whether the data can actually be collected and analyzed in the time frames proposed. Focusing discussions about data at the local level on these three key features of the evaluation process has helped guide local data collection. It has also helped to inform the national evaluation team about issues that are most relevant at the local level.

Logic Models and Indicators at the National and Local Levels

The underlying model for the Fighting Back program guided data collection at the national level (see Figure 5. 1). A community context defined by high levels of AOD use and harm leads to the motivation to develop comprehensive,

Figure 5.1. Fighting Back Logic Model

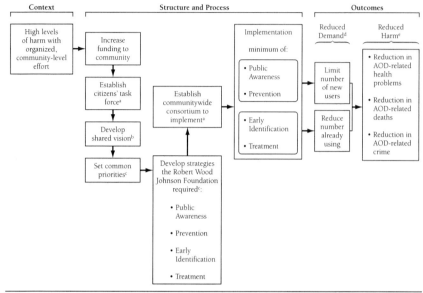

[a]From *Call for Proposals* (p. 6) (parents, clergy, tenant groups, business and commercial leaders, health professionals, school officials, judges, police, and others).

[b]From Jellinek and Hearn (1991, p. 81). Examples of shared vision might be whether to deal with substance abuse directly or with underlying causes.

[c]From *Call for Proposals* (p. 5) and Jellinek and Hearn (1991, p. 80). Priorities might be to target children, young adults, parents, or inpatients or outpatients, for example. If shared vision is to focus on underlying causes, then the effort might target the environment and other community needs.

[d]From *Call for Proposals* (pp. 5–6) and Jellinek and Hearn (1991, p. 79).

[e]From *Call for Proposals* (p. 5).

communitywide strategies to reduce demand for AOD, and thus reduce use and harm. Figure 5.2 focuses on the elements of this model that are central to the national data collection. Demographic data were used to develop a comprehensive picture of each community context. These were embellished with in-depth ethnographic studies in six of the Fighting Back communities. Further information about community context can be derived from the household survey, which includes perceptions of neighborhood, crime, attitudes and norms about drug use, and visibility of use and sales. These data, however, were not available prior to our initial involvement in 1995. Thus, they can be used only to assess community context after implementation. Data on reduced demand, in terms of the rates of new users and existing users, can also be inferred from the household survey, as can several measures of harm. The survey data should converge with other measures of harm indicated by standardized measures such as crime and mortality.

At the local level, data collection and analysis developed in a similar manner, but without the focus on standardized measures that could be uniformly collected across many sites. Sites focused on the program activities and goals that were most likely to yield significant change by the next refunding period. Examples of the types of data that communities chose to examine and the relationships of these data to the underlying model of the program are depicted in Figures 5.3 and 5.4.

Figure 5.3 depicts a logic model and indicators for a community whose local data collection mirrors the national evaluation. It proposes to use data from the National Household Survey and from schools for indicators of reduced demand. For indicators of harm reduction, it proposes police arrest data for those arrests coded as AOD related as measures of harm. The community also

Figure 5.2. National Evaluation Measurement Model

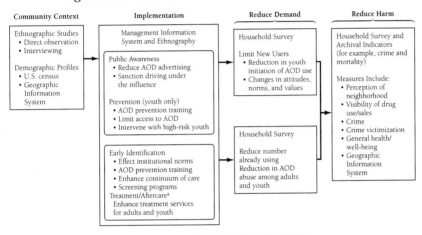

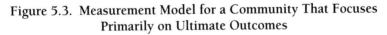

aThe household survey includes assessments on treatment and aftercare.

Figure 5.3. Measurement Model for a Community That Focuses Primarily on Ultimate Outcomes

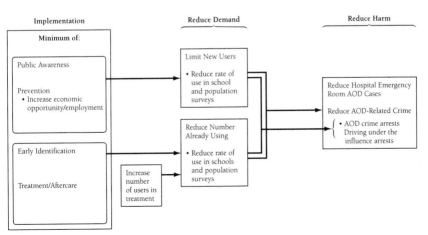

Figure 5.4. Measurement Model for a Community That Combines Ultimate and Intermediate Outcomes

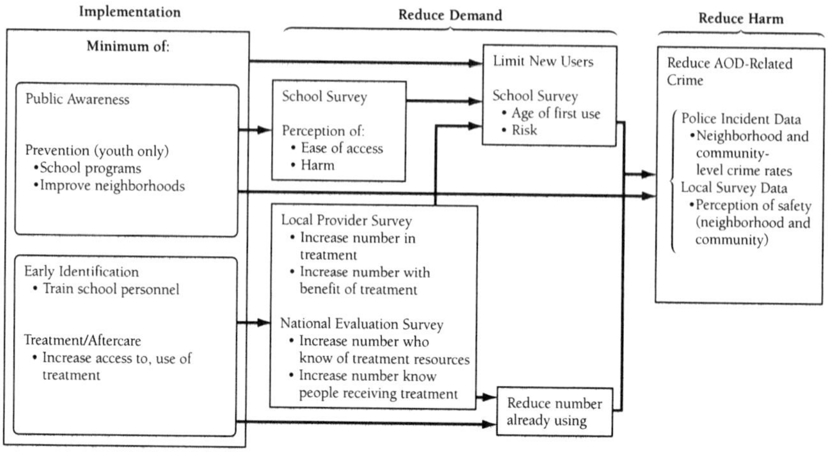

proposes that these activities will result in a greater number of people receiving treatment. This is depicted as a mediating variable between program implementation and reduced rates of people using AOD. Several different sources are proposed to estimate the number of people in the community receiving treatment, including reports of state-funded treatment slots, raw data from drug court records, and possibly estimates derived from the National Household Survey. This community also proposes the unemployment rate as a marker of success, in that increasing economic opportunities for residents should prevent substance abuse. Although employment is viewed as an element of prevention implementation, the community may choose to narrow the measurement of employment rates to those in treatment. In that case, the indicator might be better characterized as a positive outcome of treatment rather than a measure of prevention.

In the other example of local data (see Figure 5.4), the community proposes a greater number of measures that represent the mediating variables between program implementation and the ultimate outcomes of reductions in demand and harm. There is also a greater mix of data collected both locally and by the national evaluation. Prevention activities occur for the most part in schools, and school surveys are proposed to obtain the primary effectiveness data. School programs are expected to change youth norms regarding use, in particular their attitudes about perceived harm and availability. Changes in attitudes should result in reduced rates of use, as well as reduced rates of youth at risk for problem AOD use. This community's overall strategy also includes an environmental strategy focused on improving deteriorating neighborhoods. The effectiveness of these efforts will be reflected in rates of crime and perceived safety. Crime rates will be based on police incident data, and perceived safety will be based on a local survey conducted by those involved in the neighborhood intervention. These data should converge with household survey data on crime victimization and perceived safety in the neighborhood. The community also proposes to measure efforts at early identification and referral, as indicated by the number of school personnel trained. Increased access to and utilization of treatment services should be reflected in increased rates of people in treatment, which will be assessed based on a one-day sample of treatment providers' records. Although the site does not address the ultimate outcomes of communitywide decreases in AOD use and harm, the sources of data represented in this model should reflect steps toward these ultimate outcomes.

Analysis Across Local Assessment Models

These examples represent various compromises on validity to obtain maximum utility. Ideally, the national evaluation team will integrate local assessment models into the test of the underlying program construct, perhaps using meta-analytic techniques. Such a synthesis cannot be accomplished, however, without first taking into account limitations to the conclusions that can be drawn from locally collected data. Some elements of local evaluation designs may not be feasible. The strengths and weaknesses of the local data plans are best described in terms of the three key principles of validity, utility, and feasibility.

Validity. The most common problem across local data plans is a lack of fit between the program designs and the predicted outcomes. The lack of fit is an internal validity concern. Randomization was not possible at the local level, and in very few instances can comparison communities be studied. With the lack of randomization and control groups at the local level, issues of conclusion validity become a greater concern. And there is substantial variability in the degree to which the measures that have been selected reflect the program goals and activities.

Difficulties in operationalizing of constructs are shown in two areas: the ambiguous relationships among stated goals, activities, and predicted outcomes and the tendency to identify "measures" that refer to program activities rather than outcomes. For example, one community proposes to "expand treatment." Its measures of treatment expansion include rates of AOD-related hospital emergency cases, the number of health care workers trained in identification and referral, participation in aftercare services, and rates of AOD-exposed births. Each of these measures is unclear as a measure of treatment expansion. A more direct measure of whether the community has succeeded in expanding treatment would be the number of treatment slots available and whether these slots are filled by patients referred from the systems with which the community is working. Rather than focusing on hospital emergency cases, the goal of the hospital training is to get more people into treatment. Thus, a measure of the treatment services that are available, the number of people in treatment, and from where they have been referred might better reflect success in expanding treatment.

This is perhaps an extreme example of a situation in which there is a disjunction between construct and measurement. The measures in this case might still be useful, but for purposes other than the intent to measure treatment expansion. In many cases the measures reflect subgoals, or steps toward the ultimate goals. In many of the sites, however, there appears to be some confusion regarding how best to differentiate between subgoals and ultimate goals and how to incorporate the subgoals into the data plans. If the measures were operationalized in a manner that more directly corresponds to the goals or if the links to the goals were better explained, the utility of these data would be clearer.

Problems of valid measurement are also common. For example, another community proposed to examine the primary indicators of youth-related outcomes based on school survey data. For the past two years, the Fighting Back program has administered the school's substance use survey, with technical help from the national evaluators. For quite some time, the community has used the observed rates from these surveys to assess drug problems among youth. However, the survey design of these data has changed over time. Markedly different samples were drawn for each year, perhaps because of how informed consent was sought. Our involvement has led the community to modify both the way that the data are analyzed across time and the method for data collection. In this case, our focus on validity was useful to the local community and the school board.

Utility. As highlighted by the example, correspondence between measures and underlying constructs presents several problems in the interpretation and use of the data. One problem that affects the utility of the data is how proximal or distal the measures are to program activities. Another is the direction and specificity of expected effects.

Distal Versus Proximal Outcomes. The closer the unit of measure is to the actual activity, the more likely it is that the outcome will be sensitive to changes that occur as a function of that activity. Thus, communities that have more proximal outcomes are in a better position to demonstrate success than are communities that focus on distal outcomes. For example, one community proposed that its activities will result in significant changes in rates of youth and adult AOD use (as measured by surveys), rates of AOD-related crimes, and drunk driving. All of these reflect the ultimate outcomes originally expected of successful Fighting Back programs. However, they are not directly related to the specific activities occurring in the community. This community focuses on increasing AOD identification and referral to treatment at entry points into community systems, including schools, courts, hospitals, and police. Yet no measures are proposed at any of these entry points. Also, there is no measure of the community's primary goal: the identification and provision of services to substance abusers who come through the community systems.

In contrast, another community clearly distinguished between distal and proximal outcomes. Part of the plan for local data includes distal outcomes of program success that would be monitored but not used to evaluate progress toward these ultimate outcomes. Another part of the plan includes measures that more directly reflect program activities in the areas of neighborhood revitalization, treatment utilization, and youth prevention. These outcomes indicate the steps toward achieving the ultimate outcomes. There are still some questions regarding the utility and validity of the measures, but in general the measures clearly are more closely linked to the program activities than they are in other sites.

Direction and Specificity of Predicted Effects. All communities propose either to increase or decrease outcome measures, but the predicted outcomes are often opposite to what would be expected as a result of their program activities. For example, several communities propose to decrease the rate of hospital emergency cases that are alcohol or drug related. Yet in many of these communities, significant resources are invested to train hospital staff to identify and refer cases. In the long term, if the program is successful (and this is what is needed to reduce harms from substance abuse), then indeed one might expect a decreasing rate of hospital cases that are substance abuse related. The assumption of current training programs, however, is that many cases are unidentified. Thus, in the short term (at least the next one to two years), the number of cases that are identified as alcohol or drug related should increase and be a marker of program success, not failure. Conversely, with this measure alone, an observed decrease in the rate of emergency cases that are alcohol or drug related is meaningless. This could occur because staff and others have not been effectively trained or because the problem has been reduced. Without measures of the problem (overall rates of substance abuse) as well as the effectiveness of the training (for example, evidence that staff members are not underreporting cases), it would be hard to discern what a decrease would mean.

Crime data represent another outcome measure that is predicted to be opposite in direction to what might be expected. Many communities propose to decrease the rate of crimes that are alcohol or drug related, yet work with area police units should result in an increased likelihood that cases are identified as AOD related. Conversely, a decreased rate of such crimes just as likely reflects police attitudes and policies instead of progress on the problem. It would be helpful if there were a way to document police enforcement and identification process or to converge reported crime data with crime victimization surveys and the visibility of drug sales in the neighborhood, obtainable from the National Evaluation Survey. One problem, however, is that the focus of crime problems has shifted from the general idea of crimes as community harms (reflected in homicide, assault, and burglary rates) to only AOD-related crimes. This shift narrows operationalization and causes inconsistent coding from site to site, making it difficult for communities to use the national survey for converging data. It is standard at the national level to examine Uniform Crime Reports (UCR) index crimes in combination with the Crime Victimization Survey, but if sites examine only AOD-coded crimes or incidents, convergent validity is nonexistent. Similar problems apply to other measures included in local data plans.

Feasibility. Feasibility reflects two issues: whether the data are possible to collect and interpret and whether the data are likely to yield significant change in the time period under investigation even if the site is completely successful at program implementation. Data the community would like to report cannot always be collected and analyzed, several communities propose to report data that do not exist, and other proposed data do not take a standard form that can be analyzed for change across time. Most communities have difficulty collecting treatment data, as well as rates of those in need who are receiving treatment. Some propose to estimate the rate based on the National Evaluation Household Survey data. Others prefer a census of all people in treatment and have rejected a survey estimate. Although some standard data exist about publicly funded treatment slots, none are available for private facilities. Rather than modifying their approaches, some communities have pursued primary data collection on their own—for example, by conducting one-day samples of those in treatment among all providers in their communities. Although these efforts will surely yield counts of people in treatment, the validity of the data and their reliability are yet to be determined. In addition, comparisons across time will be difficult since these sources of data are not available for periods before the intervention started.

The second problem is most obvious in instances in which the site proposes to report low-frequency outcomes, such as mortality rates or drug-exposed births. The national evaluation thoroughly investigated several sources of data, such as mortality and fatal vehicle crashes, and concluded that the rates of occurrence were too low for there to be sufficient power to detect significant changes across time (Beveridge and others, 1997). Thus, communities were dissuaded from including such measures, but this did not deter some who perceived that the data would be useful to examine even if they were not statistically reliable (such as rates of AOD-exposed births).

Strengths and Weaknesses of the Joint Evaluation Strategy

Conducting a community-level evaluation study is one of the most complex challenges that evaluators face (Connell, Kubisch, Schorr, and Weiss, 1995). The time frame for hypothesized change is long, the number of units that can be studied is small, the theoretical constructs are complex, and some of the most important effects may be obscured by other changes taking place. By developing a joint focus on outcomes common to many program communities and outcomes of interest to individual communities, we have tried to address many long-standing concerns about evaluation. The approach would seem to combine features of the experimental and stakeholder approaches. Nevertheless, it is difficult to determine whether the strategy is effective and whether it will improve the quality and usefulness of the evaluation.

The strengths of the joint strategy have been implicit in the discussion of how the national and local data plans were implemented. For national evaluation purposes, the joint strategy permits the collection of cross-site data that can be easily compared to address the ultimate (distal) program goals. At the same time, the evaluators make their data available for local use, tailored to a particular site. They also work with local staff to develop measures sensitive to the unique situation of the community. To the extent that national and local data can meet the criteria of validity, utility, and feasibility, the findings can help to shape both national policy and local implementation.

Different Perspectives. In theory, the model incorporates the scientific requirements of evaluation, along with a utilization focus. In practice, however, the model may be difficult to implement because of the particular outcomes that are reported. A validity-driven study design applies stringent criteria to the measurement of program outcomes and is undoubtedly conservative in concluding that there are program effects (Rindskopf and Saxe, 1998). Although one can adjust the probability of a Type 1 versus Type 2 error, the scientific bias is toward accepting the null hypothesis. As evaluators have long noted, however, this creates a gulf between the perspectives of evaluators and program staff (Weiss, 1977). As an evaluator, one is inherently skeptical; as a program developer, one is enthusiastic about the intervention.

The national evaluation (mostly surveys of drug use and attitudes) has not yet demonstrated that Fighting Back communities achieved significant reductions in drug use (Beveridge and others, forthcoming; Rindskopf and Saxe, 1998; Saxe and others, 1997). This is particularly evident when sophisticated multilevel analytic models are used to contrast target communities with comparison communities. The findings contrast with the enthusiasm of local staff, who see daily evidence of their successful work. They see the individuals who are affected directly by their programs and are beneficiaries of changes in policy that Fighting Back brought about.

Some program staff have suggested that the national evaluation, because it views the communities from "40,000 feet," cannot see the positive impact of the program. Only when viewed from "Main Street" can one see how lives are transformed by the communitywide effort to reduce demand for illicit drugs. The problem is that having an impact on just those people one can see is not the goal of the program. In fact, evidence suggests that the visibility of drug sales and use is not an indicator of underlying patterns of use (Saxe and others, 1997). The program theory is that a communitywide effort is necessary to reduce communitywide levels of drug use and abuse. Thus, although the Main Street view is an important indicator of whether the program is making progress, the desired outcome goes beyond success with small groups of people.

The key question becomes how to scale up an intervention so that it can affect the overall rates of drug and alcohol problems. A delicate balance needs to be struck between different views of the achieved outcomes. The local view is necessary as a leading indicator, while the national data are the distal indicators sought by those who funded the program and those interested in the generalizability of the program strategy for other communities. A key issue is for both the national and local stakeholders to see the advantage of the others' perspective.

Between Ideal and Real. It is not sufficient to see the value of the other perspectives or to maximize the utility of data. Unfortunately, that which would be most useful is often invalid or infeasible to collect. All sources of data have limits to their validity. That is true for surveys of drug use (Beveridge and others, forthcoming) and local indicators of the harms associated with drug use. To be sure, in some cases it is possible to collect better data, but the cost may be prohibitive (as in the case of in-person household interviews). What seems important is to work toward balance among the three principles of validity, utility, and feasibility.

Balancing these principles involves strategic decisions about what data to collect and careful allocation of resources. With some demonstration programs, for example, it does not make sense to use an experimental design and extensive outcome-oriented measures. Particularly when the issue is whether the program idea is feasible, the research questions may not be suitable for this type of assessment. Such outcome data may not have utility in this context. Similarly, it may not be worthwhile for a local community to invest heavily in a data gathering system—even if the questions are outcome oriented—if the data cannot be gathered in a valid way. Thus, for example, it might be important to know if fewer crimes are committed as a result of new drug policies, but the collection of such data is dependent on the attitudes of both community residents (who report crimes) and police (who receive reports). Unless a valid system can be developed to collect such data, the investment is not worthwhile.

Few communities have the capacity or expertise required for primary data collection or analysis of secondary data sources. Although developing such capacity is probably useful, it can be done only over time and should probably be seen as part of a system of accountability and continuous quality improvement (Bickman and Noser, forthcoming; Wandersman and others, 1998). Where communities have collected primary data, the diversion of funds from program activities may not have been wise. Fighting Back communities have been encouraged to form local CEWGs so that the demands on local staff would be minimal, but this has yielded mixed levels of support. Each community was to have a full-time staff person who would coordinate the local data collection and analysis efforts. Although some Fighting Back communities have such a person, the task has proved difficult. The local data collectors have struggled to integrate their reporting on program success in a way that is acceptable to both their funders and the community group. Also, in sites without a full-time staff person that rely on local CEWGs, the community group acts more like an outside consultant with a narrow mandate. The group does not question the utility of the data or its relation to program activities; instead it tries to figure out how to collect data.

From the initial stages of our involvement with the evaluation of Fighting Back, we have been eager to provide sites with data. In part, we wanted to maximize the utility of the data; in addition, interaction with the sites is valuable to understand their perspectives on the problem. We conducted several sessions to feed back data and provided each site with a summary of data specific to their community. We were sensitive not to provide comparisons among sites and to provide contextual information that would aid understanding. These efforts were only partially successful. In retrospect, what was clear was that only a few sites had the capacity to use the data successfully and that substantial resources would be needed to assist the others to use data.

Sharing data with the sites has been useful but raises several concerns. The first has to do with a key change in Fighting Back: data may be used to make funding decisions. Providing data creates the potential for "dueling" evaluations whereby the national evaluators and local communities each have their own analyses—and reach their own conclusions. They may become motivated to look good so as to be refunded, and ours is "to find out the truth." Moreover, a recompetition of funding based on results may be unworkable. The prevention and treatment of substance abuse is a multivariate problem. One community's context may simply prevent changes of a size seen in other communities. The data elements cannot be treated in isolation from this context.

Although designed to empower communities to use evaluation, implementation of local data collection was not entirely up to communities' free choice. Development of local data became a requirement of funding from the Robert Wood Johnson Foundation, and it is not yet clear whether all communities recognize the benefits of data about the nature of their problem and the outcomes. However, the exercise has other advantages. It may offer the same advantage as cost-benefit analysis (Office of Technology Assessment, 1980). The process of conceptualizing outcomes helps communities go beyond what they can see directly and enables them to think about planning in a different way. At the same time, it brings evaluators into close contact with the communities and requires that they think about the intervention in terms of very specific outcomes.

Healthy Tension. Kurt Lewin (1951), the progenitor of social psychology, posited that individuals hold multiple ideas in a system of tension. The relationship of national and local evaluation perspectives for Fighting Back is Lewinian, because we see the perspectives as being in productive tension. No single perspective provides the answers that will enable the development of more effective policy. Sometimes local and national perspectives will yield different conclusions. But these conclusions are not inherently in conflict; they may be the basis for improved thinking about the program.

To preserve a healthy tension, however, there must be fundamental agreement about the purpose of evaluation. For Fighting Back, these purposes are framed as principles for evaluation: validity, utility, and feasibility. Learning will be maximized if both community and national stakeholders are committed to finding feasible strategies to develop useful and valid information. The beneficiaries will be the citizens in each of the communities that have invested in the development of new programs and their evaluation.

References

Beveridge, A., and others. *Monitoring Archival Indicators of Alcohol and Other Drug Harm.* Report prepared for the Robert Wood Johnson Foundation. Waltham, Mass.: Brandeis University, 1997.

Beveridge, A., and others. "Survey Estimates of Drug Use Trends in Urban Communities: General Principles and Cautionary Examples." *Journal of Substance Use and Misuse,* Forthcoming.

Bickman, L., and Noser, K. "Meeting the Challenges in the Delivery of Child and Adolescent Services in the Next Millennium: The Continuous Quality Improvement Approach." *Journal of Applied and Preventive Psychology,* forthcoming.

Botvin, G. J. "Substance Abuse Prevention Research: Recent Developments and Future Directions." *Journal of School Health,* 1986, *56,* 369–374.

Botvin, G. J., and others. "A Psychological Approach to Smoking Prevention for Urban Black Youth." *Public Health Report,* 1989, *104* (6), 573–582.

Botvin, G. J., Baker, E., Filazzola, A. D., and Botvin, E. M. "A Cognitive Behavioral Approach to Substance Abuse Prevention: One Year Follow-Up." *Addictive Behaviors,* 1990, *15,* 47–63.

Botvin, G. J., and others. "Smoking Prevention Among Urban Minority Youth: Assessing Effects on Outcome and Mediating Variables." *Health Psychology,* 1992, *11* (5), 290–299.

Botvin, G. J., and others. "Long-Term Follow-up Results of a Randomized Drug Abuse Prevention Trial in a White, Middle-Class Population." *Journal of the American Medical Association,* 1995, *273* (14), 1106–1112.

Campbell, D. T. "Reforms as Experiments." *American Psychologist,* 1969, *24,* 409–429.

Campbell, D. T. "Methods for the Experimenting Society." Paper presented at the meeting of the Eastern Psychological Association, New York, and at the meeting of the American Psychological Association, Washington, D.C., 1971.

Campbell, D. T. *Methodology and Epistemology for Social Science: Selected Papers.* Ed. E. S. Overman. Chicago: University of Chicago Press, 1988.

Center for Substance Abuse Prevention. *Fourth Annual Report of the National Evaluation of the Community Partnership Demonstration Grant Program.* Rockville, Md.: CSAP, U.S. Department of Health and Human Services, 1996.

Chen, H., and Rossi, P. H. "Evaluating with Sense: The Theory-Driven Approach." *Evaluation Review,* 1983, *7,* 283–302.

Connell, J. P., Kubisch, A. C., Schorr, L. B., and Weiss, C. H. (eds.). *New Approaches to Evaluating Community Initiatives: Concepts, Methods, and Contexts.* Washington, D.C.: Aspen Institute, 1995.

Cronbach, L. J. *Designing Evaluation of Educational and Social Programs.* San Francisco: Jossey-Bass, 1982.

Fetterman, D. M. "Empowerment Evaluation: An Introduction to Theory and Practice." In D. M. Fetterman, S. J. Kaftarian, and A. Wandersman (eds.), *Empowerment Evaluation: Knowledge and Tools for Self-Assessment and Accountability.* Thousand Oaks, Calif.: Sage, 1996.

Fetterman, D. M., Kaftarian, S. J., and Wandersman, A. (eds.). *Empowerment Evaluation: Knowledge and Tools for Self-Assessment and Accountability.* Thousand Oaks, Calif.: Sage, 1996.

Hawkins, J. D., Catalano, R., and Miller, J. "Risk and Protective Factors for Alcohol and Other Drug Problems in Adolescence and Early Adulthood: Implications for Substance Abuse Prevention." *Psychological Bulletin,* 1992, *112* (1), 64–105.

Hunt, M. *The New Know-Nothings: The Political Foes of the Scientific Study of Human Nature.* New Brunswick, N.J.: Transaction Publishers, 1998.

Jellinek, P. S., and Hearn, R. P. "Fighting Drug Abuse at the Local Level: Can Communities Consolidate Their Resources into a Single System of Prevention, Treatment, and Aftercare?" *Issues in Science and Technology,* 1991, *7* (4), 78–84.

Lewin, K. *Field Theory in Social Sciences: Selected Theoretical Papers.* Ed. D. Cartwright. New York: Harpers, 1951.

Musto, D. F. "Historical Perspectives on Alcohol and Drug Abuse." In J. H. Lowinson, P. Ruiz, R. B. Millman, and J. G. Langrod (eds.), *Substance Abuse: A Comprehensive Textbook.* (2nd ed.) Baltimore, Md.: Williams and Wilkins, 1992.

Office of National Drug Control Policy. *The National Drug Control Strategy, 1998: A Ten Year Plan.* Washington, D.C.: Executive Office of the President of the United States, 1998.

Office of Technology Assessment. "The Implications of Cost-Effectiveness Analysis of Medical Technology," 1980.

Patton, M. Q. *Utilization-Focused Evaluation.* Thousand Oaks, Calif.: Sage, 1978.

Patton, M. Q. *Utilization-Focused Evaluation: The New Century Text.* (3rd ed.) Thousand Oaks, Calif.: Sage, 1997.

Rindskopf, D., and Saxe, L. "Zero Effects in Substance Abuse Programs: Avoiding False Positives and False Negatives in the Evaluation of Community-Based Programs." *Evaluation Review,* 1998, 22 (1), 76–92.

Robert Wood Johnson Foundation. "Fighting Back: Community Initiatives to Reduce Demand for Illegal Drugs and Alcohol (Call for Proposals)." Princeton: Robert Wood Johnson Foundation, 1989.

Saxe, L., and Fine, M. *Social Experiments: Methods for Design and Evaluation.* Thousand Oaks, Calif.: Sage, 1981.

Saxe, L., and others. "Think Globally, Act Locally: Assessing the Impact of Community Based Substance Abuse Prevention." *Evaluation and Program Planning,* 1997, 20 (3), 357–366.

Scriven, M. "Truth and Objectivity in Evaluation." In E. Chelimsky and others (eds.), *Evaluation for the 21st Century: A Handbook.* Thousand Oaks, Calif.: Sage, 1997.

Shadish, W. R., Jr., Cook, T. D., and Leviton, L. C. *Foundations of Program Evaluation: Theories of Practice.* Thousand Oaks, Calif.: Sage, 1991.

Spickard, A., Dixon, G., and Sarver, F. "Fighting Back Against America's Public Health Enemy Number One." *Bulletin of the New York Academy of Medicine,* 1994, 71, 111–135.

Stake, R. E. "To Evaluate an Arts Program." In R. E. Stake (ed.), *Evaluating the Arts in Education: A Responsive Approach.* Columbus, Ohio: Merrill, 1975.

Stake, R. E. "Program Evaluation, Particularly Responsive Evaluation." In W. B. Dockrell and D. Hamilton (eds.), *Rethinking Educational Research.* London: Hodder and Stoughton, 1980.

Tobler, N. S. "Meta-Analysis of 143 Adolescent Drug Prevention Programs: Quantitative Outcome Results of Program Participants Compared to a Control or Comparison Group." *Journal of Drug Issues,* 1986, 16 (4), 537–567.

Tobler, N. S., and Stratton, H. H. "Effectiveness of School-Based Drug Prevention Programs: A Meta-analysis of the Research." *Journal of Primary Prevention,* 1997, 18 (1), 71–128.

Wandersman, A., and others. "Comprehensive Quality Programming: Eight Essential Strategies for Implementing Successful Prevention Programs." *Journal of Primary Prevention,* 1998, 19 (1).

Weiss, C. H. "Introduction." In C. H. Weiss (ed.), *Using Social Research in Public Policy Making.* San Francisco: New Lexington Press, 1977.

Weiss, C. H. "Improving the Linkage Between Social Research and Public Policy." In L. E. Lynn (ed.), *Knowledge and Policy: The Uncertain Connection.* Washington, D.C.: National Academy of Sciences, 1978.

Wholey, J. S. *Evaluation and Effective Public Management.* Boston: Little, Brown, 1983.

Winick, C., and Larson, M. J. "75 Community Action Programs." In J. H. Lowinson, P. Ruiz, R. B. Millman, and J. G. Langrod (eds.), *Substance Abuse: A Comprehensive Textbook.* (3rd ed.) Baltimore, Md.: Williams and Wilkins, 1997.

LEONARD SAXE *is professor of psychology at the Graduate School and University Center, University of New York, and adjunct professor of the Heller School, Brandeis University. He is principal investigator for the evaluation of the Robert Wood Johnson Foundation's Fighting Back initiative.*

ELIZABETH TIGHE *is senior research associate at the Heller School, Brandeis University, where she is co-investigator on the evaluation of Fighting Back, a Robert Wood Johnson Foundation multisite, community-based substance abuse program focused on demand reduction.*

How to engage local program stakeholders meaningfully in evaluation is a continuing challenge for many community-based program evaluators. Lessons learned from a Smart Start evaluation in North Carolina are offered.

The Process of Selling a Community Evaluation to a Community: Cumberland County's Experience

Rhode Yolanda Crago Alvarez Bicknell, Joseph Telfair

Community evaluations are increasingly on the agenda of many social service initiatives. Communities are being required to conduct or participate in community evaluations as part of a grant process or in order to provide evidence of a program's impact. Yet there remains little guidance from major grantors and government agencies as to what a community evaluation is. Thus, communities are interpreting "community" and "evaluation" in a myriad of modes. This chapter offers a description of one community's struggle to define, begin, and finally embrace community evaluation.

Background

The Cumberland County Partnership for Children (CCPFC) has been working to improve the lives of and opportunities for children in Cumberland County, North Carolina, since its inception in July 1993. The partnership assembled in response to Governor Jim Hunt's Smart Start initiative: a state-funded, comprehensive, community-based initiative to help all children and their families in North Carolina. Smart Start has targeted four core areas: high-quality early childhood education, child care accessibility, child care affordability, and health and family support. In its attempt to meet the diverse scope of Smart Start, the Cumberland County Partnership has blossomed into a dynamic and varied array of programs designed to provide services to children through age five and their families.

Smart Start is a diverse initiative with many complicated levels of accountability. It is also an initiative that must function within the constraints of uncertain funding cycles that have intermittent start-up periods (within the budget year) for each contracted program. In addition, according to Cumberland County Metro Visions' 1998 publication "1998 Community Benchmark Executive Summary," Cumberland County has an extremely high birthrate with strong out-migration. Given these tumultuous conditions, as a service entity the CCPFC has become a moving target.

Levels of Smart Start Accountability

Due to the political nature of Smart Start in North Carolina, there existed three levels of evaluation accountability. The University of North Carolina at Chapel Hill (UNC–Chapel Hill) was awarded the contract to evaluate at the state level. Its responsibility was to evaluate the impact of Smart Start in the state of North Carolina as a whole. Individual county or multicounty Smart Start Partnerships theoretically were responsible for measuring the Smart Start effects at the local county level. There were no stated requirements as to how each partnership should accomplish this task. Third, all Smart Start–funded projects were required to submit detailed project-specific evaluation plans with their proposals for funding. Regardless of these multiple evaluation efforts or requirements, there remained only a vague understanding of what each community's responsibility for evaluation actually was. Often the county- and program-level evaluation requirements were ignored, with no adverse effects from the state-funding agency.

Living with Evaluation Fear

During the first year of the evaluation, there was a great deal of resistance from Smart Start–funded programs in Cumberland County. Many of the program administrators had never previously participated in evaluation (outside of performance reviews) or designed an evaluation plan for their program. Most faced their CCPFC evaluation–mandated activities with fear and misunderstanding.

Previously this community had experienced the evaluation of the Fort Bragg Demonstration Project (FBDP). The evaluation process was perceived by many in the community as negative. Since many of the Smart Start stakeholders had been involved in some capacity with the FBDP, a similar result was feared for Smart Start if it engaged in any kind of evaluation. Although much has been written on the topic, the main lesson as it pertained to this community was that the Department of Defense did not re-fund the FBDP after the evaluation report. Therefore, the Smart Start board of directors felt that if evaluation was a requirement, it must be implemented, but they did so with much trepidation, discussion, and financial support.

Through conscientious and extensive training and technical assistance, the evaluation team has been able to garner the evaluation buy-in of Smart Start–funded programs, which is crucial in providing the outcomes and impact questions that are so often asked. Currently the same program administrators are embracing evaluation as the necessary and useful process that it can be. Moreover, these partners are voluntarily approaching CCPFC for technical assistance in writing goals, objectives, outcomes, and program-specific evaluation plans.

The CCPFC has embraced the operational aspect of evaluation since the first year of the evaluation of Smart Start. The partnership uses an outcome measurement model based on the logic model process to track inputs, activities, and outputs. A multilevel evaluation scheme has been implemented, including both process and outcome measures to examine success. The evaluation coordinator, in conjunction with the CCPFC evaluation team, is responsible for implementing the evaluation plan. The CCPFC board of directors and evaluation committee monitor evaluation efforts and report results to the CCPFC to ensure that the evaluation process meets all necessary guidelines. The evaluation plan is based on the goals of CCPFC and includes a wide range of measurement instruments and data sources (such as developmental inventories, parent inventories, and observation forms). Interim reports are provided periodically so that program staff may make use of feedback to adjust the program as necessary. A comprehensive evaluation report is prepared annually.

Phase One: Limited Community Needs Assessment

The process of evaluation began for the community partnership with a needs assessment in the spring of 1994, which targeted four economically disadvantaged communities with door-to-door interviews. The goal of the needs assessment was traditional in that it attempted to ascertain the needs of a particular community. Although the Smart Start initiative targets all children, the needs assessment methodological selection process was designed to serve only poor children in Cumberland County. The report was submitted to the statewide administrating agency in December 1994. Within two months, the findings were also presented to the North Carolina governing board of the administrating agency, to little fanfare and understanding. No action was taken on the information, and no further discussion ensued. The general consensus among the partnership's board of directors and administrative staff was that they had completed the community evaluation mandate and that the findings indicated a need for Smart Start.

Then the statewide governing agency sent additional information to the local county partnership indicating that a single needs assessment did not constitute a community evaluation of the impact of Smart Start. The agency did not, however, provide specific requirements for the completion of a comprehensive local-level evaluation. To attempt to fulfill this seemingly open-ended request, the second stage of the community evaluation process began, which involved hiring a part-time evaluator.

Phase Two: The Internal Evaluator

UNC–Chapel Hill held the contract for the statewide evaluation. Because the university had data collection needs, the local partnership and the principal investigator of the state evaluation decided that a full-time evaluator–data collector would be shared. Dividing her time equally between the state and local organizations, the evaluator–data collector collected data for the state evaluation group and provided internal evaluation guidance to the local partnership. Because there was a limited understanding from the local partnership regarding what evaluation was, much less the duties of an evaluator, there was little guidance given and even less cooperation. The evaluator was seen as a necessary evil because this community was mandated to conduct a community evaluation. Neither the Cumberland County board of directors nor the state administration provided their communities with definitions or requirements of the evaluation. The internal evaluator attempted to hold joint board of director and administration meetings to begin discussion regarding the requirements and process of community evaluations, but there was little interest and limited participation.

Because of the community's lack of understanding regarding evaluation, the internal evaluator concentrated on activities that she could accomplish rather than the full breadth of what actually needed to be done. There were two main evaluation events that occurred during this period: an assessment of the partnership's goals and objectives and an assessment of the individually funded projects' accomplishments. The partnership's goals and objectives were comprehensively reviewed for attainability and measurability. As may be expected, many of the objectives were flawed on both counts. The CCPFC had, in an attempt to expedite service delivery, adopted the individual objectives of the funded programs as its objectives. Through the "goals and objectives review," it was discovered that the CCPFC retained objectives of programs that were no longer funded and with no means of accomplishing them. The recommendation from the internal evaluator was for the CCPFC and its board of directors to engage in a strategic planning session to redefine its goals and objectives.

The result of this task had a positive outcome: as the recommendation was implemented, it coincided with a new Smart Start grant application. The CCPFC held a strategic planning session involving both the board of directors and concerned members of the community, in which the internal evaluator and the 1994 community needs assessment evaluator presented information in understandable and user-friendly terms. Program monitoring information (given regardless of whether a specific project had met its goals and objectives) was also presented. The result was no change to the mission or goals, but the objectives were redefined to be slightly more attainable and measurable. There were over thirty-five new objectives.

Phase Three: The Evaluation Committee

The board of directors and administration formed an evaluation committee to attempt to resolve the remaining questions about what a community evaluation should involve, to guide in the definition of community evaluation needs, and to oversee the evaluator. The evaluation committee, which consisted of a board member and selected community members, decided, with the support of the board of directors, to redevelop the evaluation as an individual contract and to request bids from outside evaluators. With no previous experience reviewing evaluation proposals, the committee invited a professor at North Carolina State University to review three evaluation proposals, and with her approval, Cumberland County selected the UNC proposal. When the proposal was accepted, the internal evaluator resigned that position and became part of the UNC–Chapel Hill evaluation team. The proposal consisted of an extensive outcomes-based evaluation and a transitory program-monitoring evaluation. The objective was to provide program-monitoring duties to UNC–Chapel Hill for the current year, while the CCPFC prepared to provide those duties in-house thereafter.

On the administrative side of the evaluation, all activities, written materials, memos, and reports had to be approved and edited by the local administration. The evaluation became personality and administration driven due to the limited understanding of evaluations by the local partnership, the board, and the funded programs. This does not imply that the evaluation held to the principles of a participatory evaluation model; it still reflected the micromanagement model. It should also be noted that approving any evaluation expenditures during this time was an exhaustive process to both the evaluation team and the committee because there was little understanding of evaluation costs.

The committee continues to struggle in defining its ultimate purpose and gaining skills to accomplish this task. It is important to remember that the evaluation committee consists of community laypeople who were asked to serve on the committee; their evaluation information base and expertise are very limited. We believe that asking a group of laypeople to review evaluation proposals and methodology can be counterproductive. Nevertheless, the committee remains in existence, although with a straggling attendance.

Phase Four: Technical Assistance

The fourth key factor in selling a community evaluation to this community was technical assistance. The importance of having provided comprehensive and frequent technical assistance to the board, administration, community, and individually funded programs cannot be overestimated. The evaluation team provides technical assistance at all levels.

There are four evaluation workshops required for all Smart Start–funded projects: writing measurable goals and objectives, writing a simple and attainable project-specific evaluation plan, gaining an understanding of the difference between outputs and outcomes, and documenting program successes and failures. In addition, all individually funded programs receive one-on-one technical assistance with the evaluation. At least two individual evaluation sessions are scheduled with all funded projects. One of the sessions centers on the project-specific evaluation report compiled from all evaluation and program-monitoring information gathered for the previous fiscal year. The report is reviewed by the program's administration and management, with a member of the evaluation team, a meeting during which the meaning and ways to use the information are discussed. The topic of the second one-on-one session depends on the needs of that funded project.

At the board of directors level, an evaluation report is given at every board meeting. This requirement has been implemented only since 1998 and has been very successful. A full update is given on evaluation activities as well as a synthesis of any evaluation reports and their findings. The evaluation reports are condensed into a PowerPoint presentation, lasting ten to fifteen minutes, by one of the members of the evaluation team and presented to the board of directors. This process has greatly increased the utilization and support of evaluation information.

After evaluation reports are presented to the board of directors, the CCPFC hosts community sessions to present the information contained within these reports. The information sessions are open to the public and advertised in the local newspaper. The goal is not only to inform the community about how Smart Start is doing in their county, but to educate them on the importance of collecting information.

It has been primarily through this major technical assistance effort that Cumberland County has begun to understand the importance of evaluation and begun to heal from previous disruptive evaluation efforts.

Phase Five: The Present

The CCPFC has moved from an agency that shelved all evaluation reports to one that values evaluation in all aspects of project and funding decision making. It has incorporated an extensive program-monitoring component, a needs-assessment component, an evaluation technical assistance component, and an outcomes evaluation component. The board of directors in particular has been highly supportive of designing a comprehensive evaluation model that not only builds the capacity of the partnership to make sound outcomes-based funding decisions, but builds the capacity of the individually funded programs to conduct and use program monitoring and evaluation information.

The CCPFC has recently engaged in an extensive countywide needs assessment consisting of five hundred face-to-face interviews with families who had children up to five years of age from all zip codes in Cumberland County and nineteen topic focus groups with a total of two hundred participants. That information, along with a study investigating the complex relationship between working and child care, extant county data review, and program-monitoring information, was used in comprehensive multiday and multigroup strategic planning sessions. The result was a two-year strategic plan written in attainable and measurable terms.

The CCPFC has begun to implement an Evaluation Assistance and Program Monitoring Component (PETAC). PETAC will provide technical assistance to Smart Start–funded agencies in other counties in North Carolina that are interested in applying evaluation methodologies to their programming, to include general program evaluation services, technical assistance, and evaluation workshops.

Lessons Learned in Selling Community Evaluations

For evaluators to "sell" the art and science of evaluation to those in community settings, several key lessons from the experiences presented here should be kept in mind. These lessons include the following:

- A community evaluation is a developmental process that cannot be rushed. The evaluators must develop an evaluation culture within the designated community.
- Garnering understanding and support of community evaluations will be greatly simplified if the stakeholders, participants, and funders of evaluation can gain a concrete understanding of the utility of evaluation information.
- The evaluator needs to include boards of directors, administrations, funded projects, other community stakeholders, and evaluation participants in all phases of the evaluation process.
- In order for community evaluations to be successful, there must be extensive technical assistance to teach the importance of evaluation to the community: what it is, how to do it, and how to use the information.
- The political, local, and state environment will heavily influence the support that community evaluations will get.
- Review the funding agencies' past experience with evaluation.
- There are many blind alleys in conducting community evaluations, and they vary by community. Evaluators must expect them all to apply to their community evaluation and be pleasantly surprised if they do not.
- Always remember that not everyone will value evaluation, regardless of how much inclusion, empowerment, and technical assistance is provided.

RHODE YOLANDA CRAGO ALVAREZ BICKNELL is evaluation consultant for Cumberland County (North Carolina) Smart Start.

JOSEPH TELFAIR is associate professor in the Department of Maternal and Child Health, School of Public Health, and director, Division of Social, Health Services and Community-Based Research, within the Comprehensive Sickle Cell Center, School of Medicine, at the University of Alabama at Birmingham.

A framework for the evaluation of health and human service programs in community settings is proposed and used to critique how well the chapters in this volume advance community-based program evaluation.

Framing the Evaluation of Health and Human Service Programs in Community Settings: Assessing Progress

Abraham Wandersman

Given the social play of the 1990s, evaluation of health and human service programs in community settings (EHHSPCS) is likely to be a high-growth sector for program evaluation. In this chapter, I assess how this volume furthers our understanding of evaluation of health and human service programs in community settings, including the roles that evaluators can play. I do this by framing some key dimensions of EHHSPCS and briefly assessing how these chapters contribute to this framework.

Key Dimensions of Evaluating Health and Human Service Programs in Community Settings

In a thoughtful chapter on the coming transformations in evaluation, Chelimsky (1997) describes three perspectives of evaluation: evaluation for accountability (for example, the measurement of results), evaluation for development (for example, the provision of evaluative help to strengthen programs and institutions), and evaluation for knowledge (for example, the acquisition of greater understanding of a specific domain).

In EHHSPCS, we are interested in obtaining all three: do the programs achieve results, how can we strengthen the prevention and treatment programs and the capacity of program personnel to evaluate and improve their own programs, and what types of health and human service programs work well with what types of problem areas in what types of populations? It would be highly limiting to choose one purpose. The field of EHHSPCS needs to answer all three types of purposes.

Although Chelimsky discusses the different emphases and complementary relationships among the three perspectives, it is possible to achieve progress in answering more than one purpose with a single, rich approach—if the purposes are thought of in dimensional terms. For example, the goal of empowerment evaluation is to improve program success. By providing program developers with understanding and tools for assessing the planning, implementation, and results of programs, program personnel have the opportunity to improve planning and implementation of programs and thereby increase the probability of achieving results.

Dimensions for Assessing Progress in EHHSPCS

Exhibit 7.1 lists dimensions that can be used to assess what we know from a particular study and eventually what we can know from a synthesis of evaluations in EHHSPCS. The dimensions are the beginning of a framework and can be used to frame assessments of progress in EHHSPCS.

Some of these dimensions are familiar to evaluators of all programs—for example, the stage of evaluation, goals of evaluation, tools, and use of results. These have been addressed by evaluators as diverse as Suchman (1967), Rossi and Freeman (1993; Rossi, Freeman, and Lipsey, 1999), and Cronbach (1982). However, the framework is somewhat different for community settings, because dimensions specific to these settings transform the issues. For example, a major issue in the domain of EHHSPCS concerns the roles of community stakeholders (including staff, volunteers, and participants) and evaluators in program evaluation. Typically there is a contrast in approaches. In participatory, collaborative, and empowerment evaluation, the evaluator tends to work closely with the program personnel, who play a large role in conducting the evaluation, while in more traditional approaches the evaluator emphasizes a neutral role and conducts the evaluation himself or herself.

Other dimensions of this framework come from the defining characteristics of community settings. Evaluations in community settings often focus on the capacities of the groups addressing the problem. For example, special consideration is often given to the organizational capacity of the health or human service program provider under study. Sometimes the direct or indirect result of programming or of evaluation can be changes in the functioning and capacity of the provider—capacity for both programming and evaluation. Although organizational capacity can certainly be a feature of evaluation in many settings, it is the focus on community capacity that truly distinguishes much of this work.

Assessing Progress: Commentary

In this section, I use the dimensions just set out to assess how the chapters in this volume contribute to EHHSPCS. I was asked to comment on the chapters after they were written. Therefore, the authors were not aware of these

Exhibit 7.1. An Emerging Framework for Evaluation of Health and Human Service Programs in Community Settings

Dimensions	Emerging Typology
Stakeholder roles	Program personnel: Closely involved in conducting evaluation Not involved in conducting evaluation Other community stakeholders? Close relationship with evaluator Distant or neutral relationship with evaluator (same issues)
Stage of evaluation	Developing goals Data collection Stakeholder involvement by stage; clarity of goals, activities, Data analysis logic model; feasible designs and available data Data interpretation
Goals of the evaluation	Assess outcomes and impacts of a program Improve program success/increase Continuous quality improvement. Add new program components. results over past performance Increase capacity and develop program skills Program personnel skills in planning, implementing, and evaluating Improve knowledge of what works for whom Develop program theory, database of results, dissemination strategies

Tools, instruments, and methods	Appropriate to program and evaluation stages:
	  • Planning
	  • Implementation
	  • Evaluation
	  • Continuous quality improvement
	Different types of methods can be used:
	  • Qualitative (such as focus groups)
	  • Quantitative (such as surveys, MIS)

Use of results	Future funding and resource allocation Program utility Program improvement
Organizational capacity of health or human service program provider	Organizational functioning Changes in management, policy decisions, types of programs offered Evaluation capacity Changes in how the organization monitors program planning, implementation, evaluation Programming capacity Changes in how programs are planned and implemented

Community capacity	Capacity of community residents to mobilize for: • Prevention and health promotion activities
	   • Endorsement, resource donation, advocacy
	Capacity of community residents for evaluation • Participate in planning and conduct
	   • Interpret results and use them

Funding sources	Federal State National Foundation Community Community foundation, United Way, and so on

dimensions, and I am not using them to judge their work in a post hoc framework. Rather, I am using the dimensions to help me frame how a chapter helps us progress in our knowledge of EHHSPCS.

Chapter 1: The Community as Client. When I had an opportunity to present a workshop on evaluation to new Drug Free Communities grantees in 1998, I compared this experience to a workshop I presented on evaluation to new community partnership grantees in 1991. There were several major differences, including that in 1998 virtually all project directors recognized that program evaluation was important, were eager to learn about evaluation, and were very interested in science and best practices and in accountability. This demonstrated to me a dramatic shift from the 1991 attitudes in which project directors generally viewed evaluation as a necessary adjunct to funding but separated from practice and the province only of the evaluators. This chapter by Telfair and Leviton describes in community stakeholders' own words the importance they attach to evaluation. The leaders whom Telfair and Leviton interviewed are indicators of a growing movement in community programs to understand that evaluation can be helpful to the program personnel and to program functioning, as well as being necessary to satisfy funders.

In relation to the dimension of goals of the evaluation, the community leaders clearly state the importance of evaluation for knowing whether the program works and for improving the program. It is clear from this chapter (and the other chapters in this volume) that the relationship between the evaluator and the community stakeholders is crucial to planning and implementing an evaluation. This chapter provides the perspective of articulate community leaders on such issues as the following: When should evaluation be done? What types of services most need evaluation? What are the characteristics of a good evaluator? What are the characteristics of a good evaluation? What is the ideal evaluation model for community health programs? What should evaluators who want to work in community health and social programs know? I (Wandersman, 1999) have proposed that we are likely to make significant advances in results-based accountability when community stakeholders, evaluators (and researchers), and funders work collaboratively to obtain results. Therefore, the relationships among these groups are key. It would be useful to complement Telfair and Leviton's approach and questions asked of community stakeholders with the same or similar questions asked of funders and of evaluators.

Chapter 2: Discovery Capacity. Business and, increasingly, health and human service programs have encouraged continuous quality improvement in their programs so that they can become more effective over time. Leviton and Schuh appear to be making a similar argument for evaluation: maintaining a discovery capacity in the evaluation of a project is likely to lead to an improved evaluation that is more informative about what really happened so that we can learn more from it for future efforts. Therefore, this chapter addresses fairly explicitly Chelimsky's third evaluation perspective: evaluation for knowledge.

By providing a number of examples of how discovery capacity illuminated processes and findings, Leviton and Schuh demonstrate the need for developing a strong program theory in EHHSPCS. Chen's (1990) theory-driven evaluation, Goodman and Wandersman's (1994) model of the problem—model of the intervention (1994), and Weiss's (1998) theory of change describe how program theory can be developed in EHHSPCS-type programs. Leviton and Schuh provide additional support about why this should happen more frequently and with greater resources.

Leviton and Schuh provide examples of discovery capacity that relate to a number of the dimensions in the framework, including discovery capacity at different stages of evaluation and the use of different methods (for example, qualitative and quantitative). There are many questions that can be raised to specify the use of discovery capacity. For example, is the purpose of formalizing the term *discovery capacity* to harness and legitimize what is naturally done by the community, is it to interest the evaluator in learning to perform it, is it to interest the funder to provide the resources for it, or some combination of these aims? These should be more clearly addressed. Another example involves the goal of evaluation and the discussion of the use of the experimental methods. The authors suggest that if the goal of the evaluation is results, the experimental method is often preferable because what various stakeholders want to know is whether there are results. Although the experimental method has some advantages in assessing results, there are many times when the experimental method is not the best or the most feasible method to assess results (a typical argument in the field of EHHSPCS). In addition, it appears to me that discovery capacity seems to offer advantages that can be informative in any type of evaluation design, although it is not likely to be given much importance in experimental designs (as addressed by Leviton and Schuh in their discussion of preordinate and responsive evaluation).

One of the areas that will need to be addressed in the future is how to use discovery capacity in an evaluation in a systematic way. Discovery capacity should not rely on serendipity as heavily as it appears to in this chapter. It is too important. A formal approach to discovery capacity needs to be developed and communicated.

Chapter 3: Evaluating Community-Based Health Programs That Seek to Increase Community Capacity. This chapter has the admirably ambitious objective of operationalizing and measuring community capacity. Community capacity seems to many evaluators, policymakers, and funders to be an elusive or ambiguous concept. By using four case examples, important progress is made in many of the EHHSPCS dimensions described in Exhibit 7.1. Qualitative and quantitative methods, involvement of community stakeholders in different stages of the evaluation, and changes in community capacity (functioning) are described. The authors probably have a wealth of material that could address some of the other dimensions—for example:

Whether and how different goals of evaluation were achieved, especially health impacts

The extent to which organizational capacity and community capacity for evaluation were enhanced (the emphasis reported is on capacity for functioning as a group of organizations or as a community)

How the results of the evaluation were used for funding and for program improvement purposes

The authors make an interesting distinction between evaluating general health programs and evaluating categorical health programs and report that they are now engaged in the latter. This will be important for our understanding the dimension of the goal of evaluation: improving the knowledge of what works for whom (Chelimsky's third perspective of evaluation for knowledge).

Chapter 4: Improving the Prospects for a Successful Relationship Between Community and Evaluator. Telfair helps us get to the heart of a major issue in EHHSPCS: the relationship between evaluator and community. As more and more programs want or are required to have evaluations, their level of preparation to engage in evaluation is critical. Telfair describes the Evaluation Pre-Screening Tool, an instrument that organizations fill out to describe their programs, goals, capacity, and motivation to evaluate. Having an instrument to put the issues on the table is helpful in addressing key points early on and in a more neutral manner than if an evaluator came in and verbally asked the questions. Answering a long series of verbal questions might lead to a more defensive stance than if the questions are asked as part of a standardized assessment of evaluation goals and preparedness. This type of instrument represents a real plus for a tool kit of EHHSPCS.

It may be that sharpening the questions in the prescreening tool to ask specifically about the framework dimensions would be helpful. For example, there was ambiguity and confusion about evaluation goals in the example of a community-based service agency serving persons with a blood disorder. In the prescreening tool, it would be useful to ask specifically about the extent to which the goals of the evaluation are to assess outcomes, assess organizational capacity or program fidelity, or obtain knowledge about home health services for a blood disorder, or some combination of these.

The prescreening tool poses a possible dilemma. As the chapter's conclusion suggests, three of four examples of using the prescreening tool led to less evaluation being performed or to an evaluation not being performed at all. Therefore, it appears that the tool has helped to bring the reality of time, capacity, and motivation more quickly into focus. This is important because of the limited time and energy of community agencies and evaluators. However, it is clear from the questions in the prescreening tool that it would take a considerable amount of time and capacity to fill out the tool. In terms of developing wider use of EHHSPCS, the program evaluation field, or at least those who promote empowerment evaluation, will need to develop tools that help build the capacity and interest of community agencies to fill out the tool in the first place.

Chapter 5: The View from Main Street and the View from 40,000 Feet. Saxe and Tighe discuss their experiences of a national evaluation of community-level interventions in multiple communities. This is a valuable addition to this collection because it comes from a very different tradition from the other chapters and describes experiences and raises new questions for

EHHSPCS. The impetus for evaluation and the initial evaluation perspective were to provide funders with an outcome evaluation of an expensive community intervention for the reduction of substance abuse. The perspective and utility of local buy-in of evaluation and use of data became very important to all parties: funder, community, and evaluator. There were important evolutions in the evaluation, and a mixed model is used and discussed in this chapter. The mixed model creatively clarifies and attempts to address typical major tensions between evaluators and communities around traditional outcome evaluation.

The chapter does use stereotypical tensions and divisions, which are generally accurate, but do not have to be true by definition. Using some of the dimensions for evaluating EHHSPCS, it appears that the authors discuss the evaluation interest of local communities, as in providing good news and maintaining funding, and the evaluation interest of the funder, as in learning whether the program worked. I propose that the goals of evaluation are, or should be, more complex. The funder is probably interested in several goals of evaluation: was the initiative successful (did the intervention communities achieve better outcomes than the comparison communities), was the evaluation useful for program improvement, and was the evaluation useful to our knowledge of community interventions for substance abuse prevention? In other words, for program theory and future funding purposes, does the approach of community coalitions work for community-level change, and what theory or policy change is proposed for the future? Similar questions can be and should be of interest to local communities so that they invest their resources appropriately. It appears to me that many evaluators and policymakers believe that local communities want program evaluation only to make them look good. Or they believe that more enlightened local communities want evaluation for program improvement purposes. Of course, this is true. Yet more and more communities want results as much as, if not more than, funders do. Increasingly, an interest in results does not have to be seen as a matter of conflict between grantees and funders. In empowerment evaluation, there is a common interest in results among funders, grantees, and evaluators, *and* they all work together to achieve results (Fetterman, Kaftarian, and Wandersman, 1996).

Chapter 6: Selling Evaluation to a Community. This chapter describes encounters that are typical of evaluators working in communities on EHHSPCS. The encounters are typified by community fear of evaluation, community motivation dictated by funding requirements, and limited evaluation capacity. The chapter also illustrates that the three perspectives of evaluation that Chelimsky described really can be mixed. The mandate for evaluation was driven by a state funding requirement for accountability (outcomes and impacts), yet the evaluation appears to have been conducted in very close relationship with the community (which Chelimsky usually designates as for developmental purposes).

It would be useful to have more information about the dimensions in the framework, such as the tools and instruments used in the evaluation process, the use of results, and organizational capacity. For example, it would be helpful to know more about the use of the results at the three levels: state, county, and project. There is some indication that the results were not used at the state level, and it is not clear what type of use (future funding, program utility, program improvement) occurred at the other levels. In relation to organizational capacity, the authors suggest a very nice growth in evaluation capacity (in which the organization was eventually able to offer evaluation assistance to other similar projects). It would also be interesting to know whether organizational functioning or prevention programming practice was improved.

Conclusion

This volume contributes a great deal to our progress in developing EHHSPCS. It joins a number of other chapters and volumes relevant to EHHSPCS (Fetterman, Kaftarian, and Wandersman, 1996; Goodman and others, 1996; Milstein, Wetterhall, and the CDC Evaluation Working Group, 1999; Rootman and McQueen, forthcoming). There is a need to assess and synthesize where we are and where we are heading. Perhaps the dimensions described in this chapter can serve as a basis for evaluating health and human service programs in community settings.

References

Chelimsky, E. "The Coming Transformations in Evaluation." In E. Chelimsky and W. Shadish (eds.), *Evaluation for the 21st Century: A Handbook.* Thousand Oaks, Calif.: Sage, 1997.

Chen, H. T. *Theory-driven Evaluations.* Thousand Oaks, Calif.: Sage, 1990.

Cronbach, L. J. *Designing Evaluations of Educational and Social Programs.* San Francisco: Jossey-Bass, 1982.

Fetterman, D., Kaftarian, S., and Wandersman, A. (eds.). *Empowerment Evaluation: Knowledge and Tools for Self-Assessment and Accountability.* Thousand Oaks, Calif.: Sage, 1996.

Goodman, R., and Wandersman, A. "FORECAST: A Formative Approach to Evaluating Community Coalitions and Community-Based Initiatives." *Journal of Community Psychology,* 1994, special issue, 6–25.

Goodman, R., and others. "An Ecological Assessment of Community-Based Interventions for Prevention and Health Promotion: Approaches to Measuring Community Coalitions." *American Journal of Community Psychology,* 1996, *24* (3), 263–274.

Milstein, B., Wetterhall, S., and the CDC Evaluation Working Group. "Recommended Framework for Program Evaluation in Public Health Practice." *Morbidity and Mortality Weekly Report: Recommendations and Reports Series.* Atlanta, Georgia, Feb. 2, 1999.

Rootman, I., and McQueen, D. (eds.). *Evaluating Health Promotion Approaches: Principles and Perspectives.* Copenhagen, Denmark: World Health Organization—Europe, forthcoming.

Rossi, P. H., and Freeman, H. E. *Evaluation: A Systematic Approach.* Thousand Oaks, Calif.: Sage, 1993.

Rossi, P. H., Freeman, H. E., and Lipsey, M. W. *Evaluation: A Systematic Approach.* (2nd ed.) Thousand Oaks, Calif.: Sage, 1999.

Suchman, E. A. *Evaluative Research.* New York: Russell Sage Foundation, 1967.

Wandersman, A. "Community Interventions and Effective Prevention: Bringing Researchers/Evaluators, Funders, and Practitioners Together to Promote Accountability." Unpublished manuscript, 1999.

Weiss, C. *Evaluation.* (2nd ed.) Englewood Cliffs, N.J.: Prentice Hall, 1998.

ABRAHAM WANDERSMAN *is professor of psychology at the University of South Carolina.*

INDEX

Back Issue/Subscription Order Form

Copy or detach and send to:
Jossey-Bass Inc., Publishers, 350 Sansome Street, San Francisco, CA 94104-1342

Call or fax toll free!
Phone 888-378-2537 6AM-5PM PST; Fax 800-605-2665

Back issues: Please send me the following issues at $23 each.
(Important: please include series initials and issue number, such as EV90.)

EV _____

_____

_____

$ _____ Total for single issues

$ _____ Shipping charges (for single issues **only;** subscriptions are exempt
from shipping charges): Up to $30, add $5^{50} • $30^{01}–$50, add $6^{50}
$50^{01}–$75, add $7^{50} • $75^{01}–$100, add $9 • $100^{01}–$150, add $10
Over $150, call for shipping charge.

Subscriptions   Please ❑ start   ❑ renew my subscription to *New Directions for Evaluation* for the year _____ at the following rate:

     ❑ Individual $65   ❑ Institutional $118
NOTE: Subscriptions are quarterly, and are for the calendar year only.
Subscriptions begin with the spring issue of the year indicated above.
For shipping outside the U.S., please add $25.

$ _____ Total single issues and subscriptions (CA, IN, NJ, NY, and DC
residents, add sales tax for single issues. NY and DC residents must
include shipping charges when calculating sales tax. NY and Canadian
residents only, add sales tax for subscriptions.)

❑ Payment enclosed (U.S. check or money order only)
❑ VISA, MC, AmEx, Discover Card #_____ Exp. date_____

Signature _____ Day phone _____
❑ Bill me (U.S. institutional orders only. Purchase order required.)
Purchase order #_____

Name _____
Address _____

_____

_____

Phone_____ E-mail _____

For more information about Jossey-Bass Publishers, visit our Web site at:
www.josseybass.com   **PRIORITY CODE = ND1**